Hysteroscopy

Hysteroscopy

Textbook and Atlas

Klaus J. Neis, Percy Brandner,
and Hermann Hepp

in collaboration with Karl Tamussino
Foreword by Jordan M. Phillips

166 illustrations, most in color

1994
Georg Thieme Verlag
Stuttgart · New York

Thieme Medical Publishers, Inc.
New York

Klaus J. Neis, M.D.
University Lecturer and Director
Obstetrics and Gynecology Clinic
School of Midwifery
Caritas-Klinik St. Theresia - Rastpfuhl
Rheinstraße 2
66113 Saarbrücken
Germany

Percy Brandner, M. D.
Obstetrics and Gynecology Clinic
School of Midwifery
Caritas-Klinik St. Theresia - Rastpfuhl
Rheinstraße 2
66113 Saarbrücken
Germany

Hermann Hepp, M. D.
Professor and Director
University Clinic of Obstetrics and Gynecology
Grosshadern
Marchioninistraße 15
81377 Munich
Germany

Karl Tamussino, M. D.
Department of Gynecology and Obstetrics
University Hospital
Auenbruggerplatz 14
8036 Graz
Austria

Frank A. Rodden, M.D., Ph. D.
401a Rio Concho Drive
San Angelo, Texas 76903
USA

Library of Congress Cataloging-in-Publication Data

Neis, Klaus J.
[Hysteroscopie, English]
Hysteroscopy: textbook and atlas/Klaus J. Neis, Percy Brandner,
and Hermann Hepp in collaboration with Karl Tamussino; foreword by Jordan M. Phillips.
p. cm.
Includes bibliographical references and index.
ISBN 3-13-799701-1. —ISBN 0-86577-489-7
1. Hysteroscopy. 2. Uterus—Endoscopic surgery.
3. Endometrium—Diseases—Diagnosis. I. Brandner, Percy.
II. Hepp, Hermann. III. Title.
[DNLM: 1. Hysteroscopy—methods. 2. Uterine Diseases—
diagnosis. 3. Uterine Diseases—surgery. WP 468 N416h 1994]
RG304. 5. H97N4513 1994
618.1 4659—dc20
DNLM/DLC
for Library of Congress   94-17573
                                                                CIP

Translated by Karl Tamussino and Frank Rodden

This book is an authorized, updated, and revised translation of the
German edition published and copyrighted 1991 by Georg Thieme
Verlag, Stuttgart, Germany.
Title of the German edition: Hysteroskopie: Lehrbuch und Atlas

© 1994 Georg Thieme Verlag,
Rüdigerstraße 14, D-70469 Stuttgart, Germany
Thieme Medical Publishers, Inc., 381 Park Avenue
South, New York, N.Y. 10016

Typesetting by Concept GmbH, D-97204 Höchberg bei Würzburg,
typeset with Quark XPress 3.2 on Apple Macintosh IIfx

Printed in Germany by K. Grammlich, D-72124 Pliezhausen

ISBN 3-13-799701-1 (GTV, Stuttgart)
ISBN 0-86577-489-7 (TMP, New York)

Foreword

Now there is a book on hysteroscopy that represents the state of the art as we know it today. Drs. Neis, Brandner, and Hepp have presented hysteroscopy in a very clear, concise, understandable way.

Whether you are a novice or a well-experienced hysteroscopist, you can greatly benefit by having this book as a source of reference and review. The text is complete; the pictures vividly demonstrate the physiology, pathology, and surgical opportunities.

The references are complete for hysteroscopy, diagnostic and operative.

The opinions expressed in this book are backed up by the authors' experience and knowledge of surgery and pathology, and of course, from having identified and treated complications, both major and minor.

Every hysteroscopist must have this book in his or her library.

Santa Fe Springs, CA 1994

Jordan M. Phillips, M.D.
Chairman of the Board
The American Association of
Gynecological Laparoscopists
Santa Fe Springs, CA
USA

Preface

The significance of imaging techniques in medicine is increasing steadily. This holds true for indirect methods, such as ultrasound or immunoscintigraphy, as well as for direct methods, such as hysteroscopy.

Modern medical technology increasingly enables us to determine the benign or malignant nature of a lesion or the extent of a malignancy early in a patient's workup. Some of this information used to be obtained only during surgery or at autopsy. These diagnostic refinements, found in all areas of medicine, have also reawakened interest in hysteroscopy, a method most gynecologists long thought they could do without.

Hysteroscopy can now give us information on intrauterine lesions that would be missed by curettage or radiological methods. Also, it is more accurate for diagnosing cancer than traditional "blind" fractional curettage.

For evaluating the endometrium or in the workup of a patient with sterility, there is hardly a question as to the proper indication for hysteroscopy. We now ask the reverse question: When is it appropriate not to perform hysteroscopy?

Hysteroscopic evaluation of the endometrium requires some skill in the macroscopic-endoscopic appraisal of the mucous membrane. With specific knowledge of endometrial morphology, it is not difficult to distinguish between benign, suspect, and malignant findings. Thus, in this book we have included a chapter on the pathology of the endometrium to meet the specific needs of the hysteroscopist.

Operative hysteroscopy has developed rapidly during the last few years, in many areas even belatedly pulling diagnostic hysteroscopy along in its wake. Dividing intrauterine septa and synechiae, resecting myomas, and resecting and ablating the endometrium have become established procedures. Many conditions of the uterus can now be treated specifically, without having to remove the entire organ. This step toward individualized treatment is in accord with many women's wishes to preserve their bodily integrity by undergoing treatments entailing minimal trauma. However, a reliable and, ideally, reversible method of transcervical tubal sterilization, which would open new dimensions in contraception, remains an unmet and elusive goal.

Interest in hysteroscopy is clearly increasing. It has become an accepted technique in hospitals and private practices, where hysteroscopes with narrow lumens now also permit outpatient hysteroscopy. Today it is a standard technique in the armamentarium of gynecology.

K J. Neis, P. Brandner, and H. Hepp   Summer 1994

Contents

History of Hysteroscopy

In his 1933 *Textbook of Gynecology,* Walter Stöckel wrote:

"Recently, experiments with hysteroscopy, such as those which were repeatedly undertaken in the past, but which never reached their goal, have been taken up again, this time with greater success. The results now are so positive that hysteroscopy must be recognized as a valuable method for diagnosis within the uterine cavity as well as for influencing tubal function."

At the time, 64 years had passed since Pantaleoni carried out the first hysteroscopy in 1869. Whereas endoscopic examinations of other organs, such as the bladder, were quickly accepted, hysteroscopy was not. Several organ-specific problems had to be solved first. These included the expansion of the uterine cavity for optimal visual inspection and the impairment of vision by iatrogenic or preexistent bleeding. Also, the hysteroscopes used by these pioneers had diameters of between 10 mm and 20 mm, and the uterus had to be maximally dilated before every examination. Light sources were weak and unwieldy.

The history of endoscopy itself began when Bozzini, a physician from Frankfurt, first considered the possibility of inspecting the body cavities of humans. In 1807 he described a "light ladder" with which the inner chambers and interorgan spaces of the human body could be illuminated and inspected. Bozzini even named the search for intrauterine tumors and the diagnosis of sterility as indications for the technique.

The first serviceable endoscope was constructed by the Frenchman Desormeaux (1865). It was conceived as a cystoscope with a diameter of 10 mm. The light source was a flame sustained by a mixture of alcohol and turpentine, and the light was guided into the shaft by a mirror. Heat and smoke were disposed of through a chimney (Figs. **1, 2**).

It was with a similar instrument that the Englishman Pantaleoni carried out the first hysteroscopy, which he reported in 1869. A 60-year-old woman with therapy-resistent bleeding was found to have endometrial polyps, which were cauterized with silver nitrate. Thus the first hysteroscopy was of therapeutic as well as diagnostic value.

The first endoscope with an optical system was described by Nitze 10 years later in the *Wiener Medizinische Wochenschrift* (1879). Through combinations of lenses, light was directed into the organ to be studied, in this case the ureter, urinary bladder, or rectum (Fig. **3**). Analogous endoscopes for hystero-

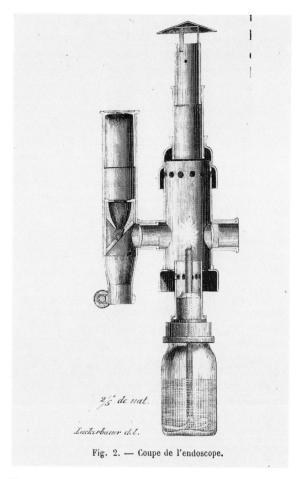

Fig. 2. — Coupe de l'endoscope.

Fig. **1** Light source of the Desormeaux endoscope with a chimney to evacuate smoke

scopy were demonstrated in 1907 by the Frenchman David, who had already constructed instruments of various widths for inspecting normal and postpartal uteri. In 1925, an American, Rubin, tried to improve the visual conditions in the uterine cavity by dilating it with CO_2. Despite favorable results, this method did not gain wide acceptance at the time.

The difficulties in distending the flattened space of the nonpregnant uterine cavity and visual impairment due to bleeding kept hysteroscopy from keeping pace with cystoscopy. Gaus (1927, 1928) expanded the uterine cavity with water and defined precisely the threshold pressure for tubal pertubation. Passage of water into the vascular system with the danger of hemolysis

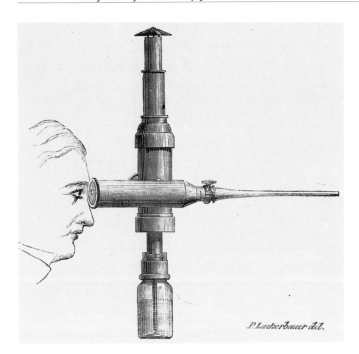

Fig. **2**   The first serviceable endoscope, designed by Desormeaux (1865)

was described as a possible complication of this method. Also, because of bleeding, vision could be sustained only by constant irrigation. The introduction of highly colloidal solutions (Menken 1969; Edström & Fernsström, 1970) was a breakthrough because these totally transparent media did not mix with blood. A disadvantage, however, was the rapid caramelization of these solutions; even slight impurities could cause considerable difficulties for the operator. Also, the instruments were damaged if not immediately cleaned with hot water.

Significant contributions to the development of hysteroscopy have been made by French (Palmer, Porto & Gaujoux, Parent, Barobot), American (Rubin, Norment), and Scandinavian gynecologists (Englund, Ingelmann-Sundberg, Silander). In the German-speaking countries Mikulicz-Radecki, Freund, Gauss, Markeschi, Menken, Lindemann, and Lübke were pioneers.

The expansion of the uterine cavity with CO_2, which Rubin had already propagated in the 1920s, was adopted and developed further by Lindemann (1971). Today, a panoramic view of the uterine cavity is the norm, and minor bleeding from mucous membranes no longer obstructs vision.

Until the early 1980s hysteroscopes with diameters of between 7 mm and 8 mm were standard. These hysteroscopes had 6-mm optics and produced well-lit panoramic pictures but were difficult to use on an outpatient basis because they required dilation of the cervical canal. But hysteroscopy soon profited from the rapid development of endoscopy as smaller and smaller optics were developed without sacrificing picture quality. Today the limited visual field and loss

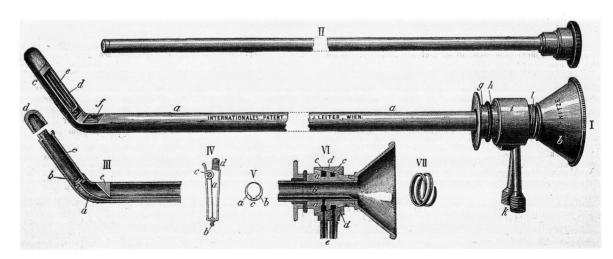

Fig. **3**   The first endoscope with an integrated optical system for light conduction, designed by Nitze (1879)

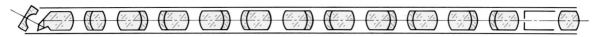

Fig. **4**   Modern standard optical wide-angle system with rod lenses

of brightness associated with small optical systems can be completely compensated by wide-angle optical systems (Fig. **4**) and effective cold-light sources.

A relatively simple mechanical instrumentarium long limited operative hysteroscopy to minor procedures such as directed biopsy, extraction of dislocated intrauterine devices, reduction of slight synechiae, and resection of pedunculated polyps. Since the second half of the 1980s the boom in minimally invasive surgery and the rapid development of laser-endoscopic and high-frequency electrosurgical technology have dramatically expanded the indications for hystero-scopic surgery. The era began with the resection of synechiae, septa, and myomas and the vaporization of the endometrium with the Nd:YAG laser (Goldrath et al. 1981, Dequesne 1987, Donnez et al. 1990). Today, operative hysteroscopy is dominated by the use of high-frequency electroresectoscopes in fluid dilation media (Neuwirth 1984, DeCherney & Polan 1983, Vancaillie 1989).

A dependable, safe, and perhaps even reversible method for tubal sterilization, a method that would advance the cause of operative hysteroscopy beyond specialized centers, has not yet been developed.

Instrumentarium

Hysteroscopes

A diagnostic hysteroscope consists of an optical system and a shaft. The shaft carries a fitting through which the dilating medium, most commonly CO_2, is introduced into the uterine cavity. This fitting generally can be opened and closed by a lever. The optical system also contains a fitting to which the fiber-optic cable from the light source is connected (Fig. **5**).

The optical system itself contains the lenses that are responsible for the device's optical properties. Thus, the field of view can be varied as can the degree of magnification (magnification depends also on the distance between objective and object).

Most manufacturers now offer a selection of objectives; all, however, use the standard diameter of 4 mm (Fig. **6**). All these instruments, regardless of manufacturer, produce views of very high quality. Even small hysteroscopes can sufficiently illuminate the uterine cavity and reveal features near the objective as well as in the depths of the uterine cavity with sharp contrast and in authentic color.

Hysteroscopes with a diameter of 2.7 mm to 3 mm are available for certain indications, such as outpatient hysteroscopy in nulliparas and chorion biopsy. These scopes are also of good optical quality, but the angle of vision and the light intensity are inferior to those of 4-mm instruments (Fig. **7**).

A cervical adapter used to belong to standard hysteroscopy equipment (Fig. **8**). After dilation of the cervical canal, the adapter was attached to the cervix and the hysteroscope was pushed forward through the adapter and cervical canal into the uterine cavity. But outpatient hysteroscopy without analgesia and dilation has shown that the tonus of the internal cervical os suffices to seal off the uterine cavity and prevent the escape of the dilation medium. Today, the adapter is hardly ever used, even in the procedures carried out under general anesthesia, unless there are anatomical changes that make additional occlusion of the cervix necessary to maintain pneumometra. Such conditions include Emmet tears, endocervical tumors, cervical extension of endometrial carcinoma, or the softening of pregnancy.

Sealing balloons, which can be pushed over the shaft (Fig. **9**), or grasping forceps with a conical seal, similar to the Schulz apparatus, are now available as alternatives to the cervical adapter. However, these systems have not proven necessary in practice, and their use is limited to the few patients with very patulous cervical canals. They are not part of the basic equipment needed for hysteroscopy.

Whereas early hysteroscopes had zero-degree forward optics, modern hysteroscopes have 25° to 30° optics. By rotating the instruments, the walls of the uterine cavity and the tubal angles can be seen without

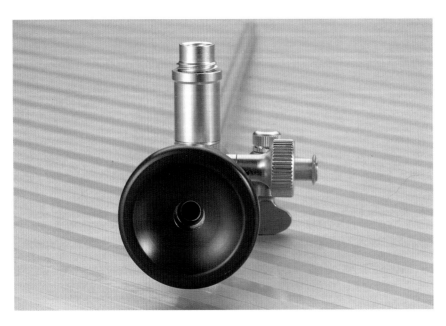

Fig. **5** Four-mm optics; the fitting for the light cable is above, that for the dilation medium at right

Fig. **6**   Small standard
hysteroscope with 4-mm
optics and a 5-mm shaft

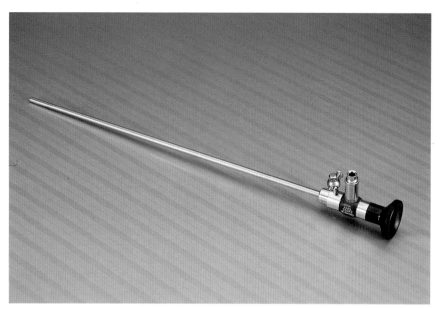

Fig. **7**   Hysteroscope with
a 4-mm shaft diameter for
special indications

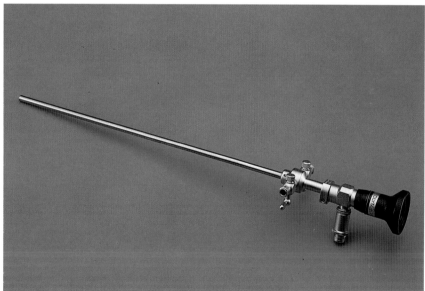

Fig. **8**   Hysteroscope with
cervical adapter

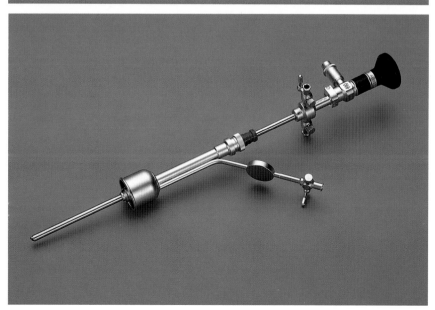

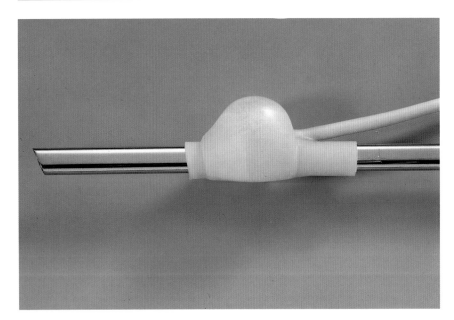

Fig. **9**   Hysteroscope end with sealing balloon

difficulty. Also, the cervical canal is easier to inspect if the optical plane is slightly inclined.

Diagnostic Hysteroscopes

Diagnostic hysteroscopes are used solely for inspection since an operating channel is unnecessary. The shaft contains only a cleft for insufflating CO_2 and is generally 5 mm in diameter. This shaft can be used in outpatient settings and before curettage under general anesthesia. An adapter is hardly ever needed. Therefore the 4-mm hysteroscope with a 5-mm shaft is the standard. Other hysteroscopes are used for special indications.

Small hysteroscopes with optical diameters of between 2.7 mm and 3 mm and working shafts of between 3.5 mm x 3.5 mm and 3.7 mm x 5 mm have been designed for special indications, such as outpatient hysteroscopy in nulliparous women, cervical canals scarred and narrowed after conization, and chorionic biopsy. Small scopes are of secondary importance in routine practice because even narrow cervical canals can easily be dilated to Hegar 5 under paracervical blockade.

Operative Hysteroscopes

Operative hysteroscopes are also equipped with a 4-mm optical system. In contrast to diagnostic hysteroscopy, at which a 25° to 30° optical system is used to obtain a good overview of the uterine cavity, operative hysteroscopy is best done with a 12° scope, which yields the best view of the surgical instrument. The shaft is 7 or 8 mm in diameter and has an operating channel through which flexible or rigid surgical instruments can be introduced and manipulated via an Albarran lever. Such instruments include biopsy forceps, grasping forceps, scissors, and tubal catheters (Fig. **10**). These hysteroscopes can be used in outpatient settings or with the

patient under general anesthesia. Whether general anesthesia is indicated depends primarily on the nature of the planned procedure.

Laser Hysteroscopes

For hysteroscopy, the neodymium:yttrium-aluminum-garnet (Nd:YAG) laser is superior to the CO_2 laser because the CO_2 laser cannot be applied through flexible glass fibers and because its beam is absorbed by even a thin film of fluid. The argon laser, which also cannot adequately penetrate fluid, is similarly unsuitable for hysteroscopy.

Because of the smoke produced by laser hysteroscopy, the 7-mm or 8-mm hysteroscope shafts designed for use with laser systems have an irrigation system that continuously feeds CO_2 into the uterine cavity through a separate channel and lets it flow out through the shaft (Baggish & Baltoyannis 1988).

Tissue dissection is done with a bare quartz glass fiber. This fiber is flexible enough to be directed accurately with the Albarran lever. In contrast to a sapphire tip, it requires no additional gas cooling (which is not permissible in the uterine cavity because it requires high flow and poses a risk of CO_2 embolism) and is comparatively inexpensive.

Resectoscopes

The resectoscopes used at hysteroscopy are modifications of the instruments designed by urologists for transurethral prostatectomy. The shaft system contains an afferent and an efferent channel for continuous irrigation, the optical system, and an operative channel fashioned so that an electrode at its tip can be moved linearly back and forth by a pistol-like grip mechanism (Fig. **11**).

Most operative hysteroscopes have a shaft 7 mm or 8 mm in diameter with a 4-mm optical system. For

Fig. **10** Surgical hysteroscope with shaft and semiflexible instruments

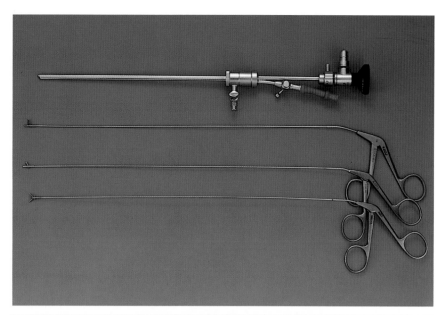

Fig. **11** Resectoscope with cutting-loop and roller-ball electrodes

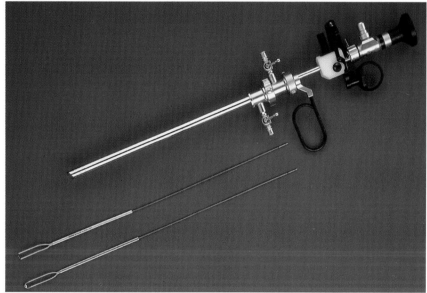

the reasons discussed above, we prefer an optical angle of 12° for operative hysteroscopy. The tip of the instrument carries a monopolar, active electrode; a neutral, grounding electrode is affixed to the patient's thigh. Three basic types of monopolar electrodes are available: cutting loops, roller balls (cylinders), and needle electrodes. The active electrode can be manipulated either actively with a Baumrucker grip, with which the electrode is outside the shaft at rest, or, more commonly, passively with an Iglesias grip, which contains the electrode within the shaft at rest.

The resectoscope uses high-frequency current. Modern systems regulate the current according to the resistance of the tissue. Tissue can be cut or coagulated depending on the amplitude and intensity of the current and on the power intensity delivered by the electrode (which depends on the shape of the electrode being used) (Fig. **12**). To avoid unintended conduction of electricity, resectoscopes can be used only in nonionic fluid distension media (discussed below).

Contact Microcolpohysteroscopes

As the name implies, contact microcolpohysteroscopes are used both in the cervix and in the uterine cavity. Magnification up to ×150 permits microscopic examination of the surface epithelium (Fig. **13**).

The principle of contact microcolpohysteroscopy is that bringing the lens closer to the object automatically increases the magnification. Placing the optical system directly on the tissue and focusing with additional lens systems further increases the magnification. The best-known contact microcolpohysteroscope, that described by Hamou (1980, etc.), permits magnifications of ×1, ×30, ×60, and ×150.

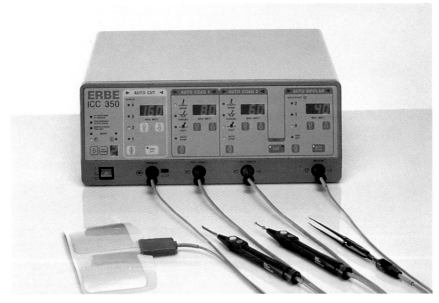

Fig. **12** High-frequency electrical generator for monopolar and bipolar cutting and coagulation automatically adapted to the resistance of the tissue

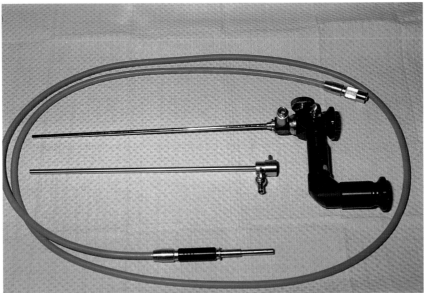

Fig. **13** Contact micro-colpohysteroscope

For contact microcolpohysteroscopy of the cervix, the tissue is first stained with ink. This is rapidly absorbed and concentrated in the nuclei of the epithelial cell (Figs. **14, 15**). The method's proponents (Scarselli et al. 1983, Mencaglia et al. 1983, Hamou 1984) claim that it permits a histologic as well as a cytologic diagnosis. In particular, the investigator should be able to define the severity and extent of cervical intraepithelial neoplasia before an operation.

In contrast, sceptics of microcolpohysteroscopy maintain that the technique cannot fulfill these expectations because, as opposed to cytology, the different grades of cervical intraepithelial neoplasia cannot be distinguished with certainty. Also, because only small areas can be observed at a time, the instrument has to be constantly repositioned to evaluate the entire cervix and cervical canal. This makes it difficult to define the location of the lesion with precision. Since contact microcolpohysteroscopy pro-

vides no reliable information beyond that provided by colposcopy and cytology, many investigators have abandoned it. The technique has not been able to establish itself in the German-speaking areas of Europe.

Autonomous CO_2 Hysteroscope

The autonomous CO_2 hysteroscope designed by Parent and Guedj consists of a 4-mm optical system with a 5-mm shaft that can be exchanged for a 7-mm shaft with an operating channel. This hysteroscope differs from others in that the light source as well as the gas inlet is integrated (Fig. **16**). The instrument was designed primarily for outpatient use and has the advantage that it can be stored in a small space. But since the light and CO_2 sources are integrated, the instrument is considerably heavier than conventional hysteroscopes and thus somewhat unwieldy.

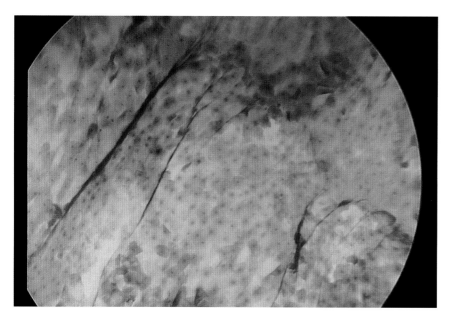

Fig. **14** Contact microcolpohysteroscopy of cervical squamous epithelium after staining with ink

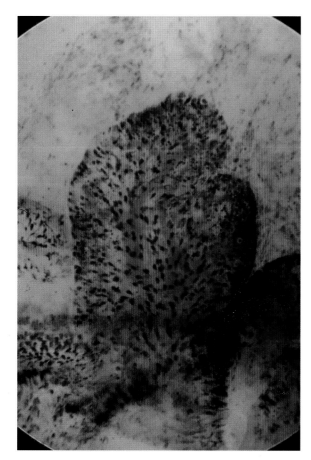

Fig. **15** Contact microcolpohysteroscopy of a papilla in the cervical canal with central vessels

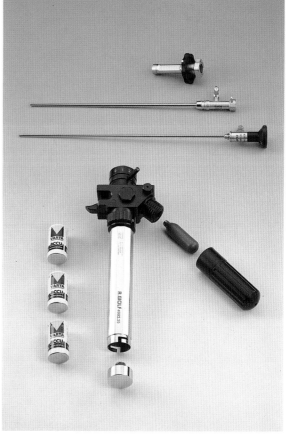

Fig. **16** Autonomous hysteroscope with integrated light source and CO_2 cartridge

Chorionoscopes

Chorionic villus biopsies can be performed with hysteroscopes designed especially for this purpose. Two systems are available; one has a lateral window that is opened only for the actual biopsy. The disadvantage of this instrument is that it has to be advanced blindly through the cervical canal into the uterine cavity and to the placenta. The tissue sample is obtained through the lateral window after aspirating the placental villi with a syringe. Chorionic villus biopsies can also be carried out under visual control with a small operating hysteroscope (shaft diameter 5 mm at most). The villi are sampled with biopsy forceps.

Both of these methods are discussed in detail elsewhere in this book (see "Operative Hysteroscopy").

Flexible Hysteroscopes

Flexible hysteroscopes, similar to the endoscopes commonly used in gastroenterology, have recently become available, particularly for operative procedures. Although they have been claimed to be superior to rigid instruments, their disadvantages are their relatively high cost and inferior optical quality due to the fiber optics (Fig. **17**).

Dilation Media

A major reason that delayed the acceptance of hysteroscopy as a routine method was that the uterine cavity is normally a flattened cleft. Inspection of the uterine cavity required a method for distending the cleft with its thick-walled myometrium, a more difficult undertaking than filling the bladder for cystoscopy. This problem was solved 100 years after the first hysteroscopy.

Today hysteroscopy can be performed with gas or liquid distension media. CO_2 is the only gas used, but a number of liquid distension media are available. For diagnostic hysteroscopy, CO_2 has proved easy and practicable for both the patient and the examiner and provides excellent visualization of the uterine cavity. In contrast, the extensive use of high-frequency electrosurgery makes operative hysteroscopy the domain of liquid distension media.

Fluid Distension Media

Irrigation fluid used to have only to provide good visibility in the uterine cavity at diagnostic and operative hysteroscopy. Today intrauterine electrosurgery is the most common indication for a fluid medium and, in addition to a clear view, the medium has to isolate the surrounding tissue from heat and electric current. Thus, a distension medium should be free of electrolytes, minimally ionizing, and conductive. To minimize the risk of a mix-up or accidental use at electrosurgery, liquids containing electrolytes (e. g., saline or lactated Ringer's solution) should be used only for purely diagnostic hysteroscopy.

A second important aspect of liquid media is their osmotic pressure. Urologists performing transurethral prostatectomies have long been familiar with a syndrome characterized by sudden blood pressure increases with bradycardia ("post-TURP syndrome").

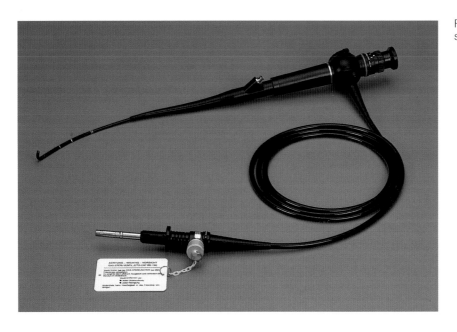

Fig. **17** Flexible hysteroscope with maneuverable tip

Further symptoms include subsequent circulatory depression, agitation, confusion, high central nervous system pressure, vomiting, shaking chills, oliguria or anuria progressing to acute renal failure, cerebral edema, and pulmonary edema (Greene 1982, Harzmann & van Deyk 1982, Zwergel 1987, Witz et al. 1993). This syndrome is caused by highly hypo-osmolar solutions entering the systemic circulation through vessels opened at surgery. The result is water intoxication with hypotonic hyperhydration, hyponatremia, and severe hemolysis (Creevy 1947). The recognition of this syndrome led to the development of osmotically corrected solutions that did not cause hemolysis. But even osmotically corrected solutions can enter the patient's circulation. The magnitude of such fluid shifts is associated with the duration of the operation, the technique used, the hydrostatic pressure in the cavity, and the size of wound surfaces. Thus, even modern dilation media entail a risk of fluid overload and water intoxication (Naber & Möhring 1973, Iglesias & Stams 1975, Trunninger 1976, Witz et al. 1993).

Currently used distension media that are osmotically corrected and free of electrolytes are Hyskon (32% dextran 70 in 10% glucose), low-molecular weight fluids (4% or 6% dextran, 5% glucose), glycine solution, and sugar alcohols (sorbitol and mannitol). Because of its high viscosity, Hyskon is not suitable for continuos-flow hysteroscopy. Also, Hyskon can caramelize and obscure vision at electrosurgical or laser procedures and can gum up instruments. Cases of anaphylactic reactions, coagulation disorders, and pulmonary edema and the adult respiratory distress syndrome have been reported with Hyskon, and it is not approved for use in all countries (Edström & Fernström 1970, Borten et al. 1983, Mangar et al. 1989, Jedeikin et al. 1990, Choban et al. 1991).

Low–molecular weight dextran solutions are obsolete because of allergic reactions. Low–molecular weight dextran and glucose solutions can gum up instrument shafts, crystallize at the electrodes, and mix well with blood to obscure vision if flow rates are too low. Also, the use of glucose solutions can affect blood glucose levels (Carson et al. 1989).

Solutions containing the nonessential amino acid glycine at a concentration of 1.5% to 2.2%, which date back to studies by Nesbit & Glickmann (1948), are used predominantly in English-speaking and French-speaking countries. These solutions are hypoosmolar and can thus cause hyperhydration and hemodilution with low sodium, albumin, and hemoglobin levels. Importantly, glycine shifted to the systemic circulation is metabolized to ammonia and oxalic acid by transamination and oxidative deamination. This can lead to deposition of calcium oxalate in the urinary tract in patients with reduced diuresis (Fitzpatrick et al. 1981). Elevated serum levels of ammonia are common if glycine is used, even in patients with normal liver function, and can lead to neurotoxic, encephalophatic sequelae ranging from mild symptoms at the end of anesthesia to agitation, vomiting, dizziness, disturbances of vision including transient blindness, and encephalopathic coma (Hoekstra et al. 1983, Roesch et al. 1983, Ovassapian et al. 1982, Ryder et al. 1984, Hahn 1988, Burkhart et al. 1990). Even if L-arginine given orally may be an antidote (Roesch et al. 1983), media containing glycine should be used with the knowledge of the potentially severe complications.

The six-carbons sugar alcohols mannitol and sorbitol have been used widely to adjust osmolarity, particularly in German-speaking countries. Mannitol, only trace amounts of which are metabolized, increases renal perfusion and diuresis. This effect, which is beneficial because it reduces the volume load on the systemic circulation, can cause blood pressure decreases after surgery. Sorbitol is rapidly metabolized to fructose in patients with intact liver function. It has a biologic half-life of only 30 minutes but is not excreted via the kidneys and thus does not have mannitol's diuretic effect (Norlen 1985). The half-life of sorbitol in the plasma is prolonged in patients with impaired liver function. Also, the endogenous fructose that is produced can cause complications in patients with impaired glucose tolerance or fructose intolerance. Finally, fructose is gylcosylated to lactic acid, so that lactic acidosis is conceivable if there is a massive shift of sorbitol into the systemic circulation.

Solutions containing both mannitol, with its diuretic effect, and sorbitol, with its rapid metabolic elimination and short half-life, make an optimal distension and irrigation fluid for operative hysteroscopy. The solutions are semi-iso-osmolar (about 178.54 mOsm/L), are diuretic but nonhemolytic, ensure good optical qualities, and do not crystallize at the electrodes. This has made the mannitol–sorbitol combination one of the most widely used irrigation fluids for urologic and gynecologic endoscopy (Madsen & Madsen 1965, Madsen et al. 1969, Hartmann 1979, Bichler et al. 1985, Zwergel 1987).

No distension medium is equally appropriate for all patients and situations. At present it seems most sensible to use a 1.5% glycine solution or a combination of 0.54% mannitol and 2.7% sorbitol.

Continuous-Flow Hysteroscopy

At operative hysteroscopy a fluid medium serves both to distend the uterine cavity and to continuously flush out bleeding arising in the surgical field (Fig. 18). The simplest way to create and maintain hydrostatic intrauterine pressure is to suspend the irrigant about 150 cm above the patient. The fluid is conducted through large-caliber tubing (as used at transurethral electrosurgery) and the shaft of the scope into the uterine cavity. If uterine distension is inadequate, the pressure can be raised by hanging the irrigant higher or by applying a pressure cuff that can be pumped up manually to the bag containing the irrigant. The flow can be increased, for example in the presence of bleeding, by opening further the efflux channel of the hysteroscope. Such a setup is simple, inexpensive, and not very prone to technical problems.

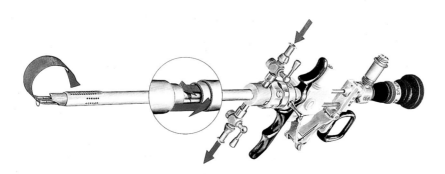

Fig. **18** Schematic representation of the continuous–flow principle in a resectoscope

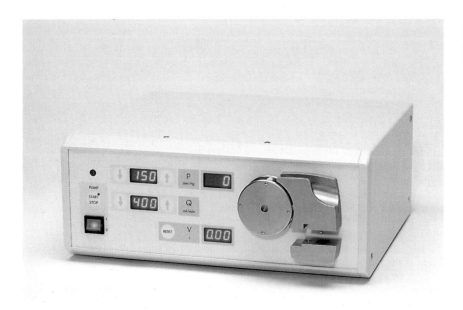

Fig. **19** Irrigation pump for fluid hysteroscopy. This pump permits presetting of pressure and flow

Irrigation pumps developed for hysteroscopy are considerably more sophisticated and expensive, albeit sometimes more exact. These electronically regulated roller pumps permit presetting of the maximum intrauterine pressure (usually at 200 mmHg) and the maximum flow rate (usually 400 mL/minute) (Fig. **19**). For safety, in addition to being electronically set to shut down at a certain pressure, these pumps have mechanical backup valves. The efflux from the uterine cavity is controlled by a vacuum pump with a negative pressure that can also be preset or, in other systems, by the operator through the efflux stopcock of the hysteroscope.

Although all pumps come with sets of large-caliber tubing, the irrigant has to pass two stenoses on its way to the uterine cavity. The first is the Luer lock on the hysteroscope and the second is the irrigation channel in the shaft. These stenoses can increase the pressure in the proximal tubing, particularly if flow rates are high. Because of the resistance between the pump and the tip of the hysteroscope, the pressure in the proximal tubing, which most pumps use as the reference value for regulating the flow, does not accurately reflect the true intrauterine pressure. Pumps are now being developed that adjust their flow rates according to the true intrauterine pressure as measured by a water column in an additional channel in the hysteroscope or by a microtip transducer at the tip of the scope. But as long as such pumps are not available, we prefer to distend the cavity using the simple and inexpensive method of suspending the irrigant and applying a pressure cuff.

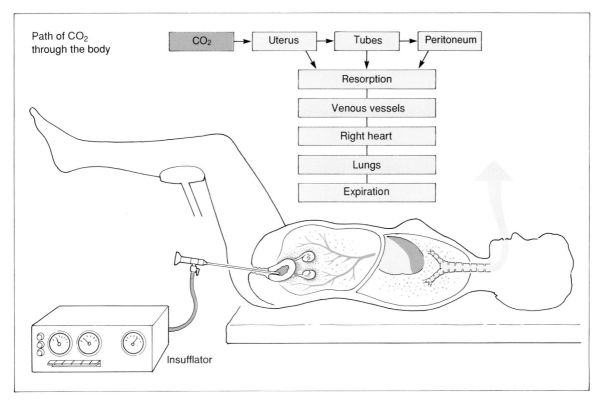

Fig. **20**   Path of insufflated CO_2 through the body during CO_2 hysteroscopy

The patient and the fluid balance should be monitored closely during the procedure to avoid the dangerous and potentially lethal complications discussed above. The patient's status can be monitored clinically if regional anesthesia is used (see also "Complications Associated with Anesthesia"). The simplest way to monitor fluid balance is to subtract the volume coming out of the uterine cavity from that introduced into it (measured by reading the volume from the pump or by weighing the container). An effort should be made to catch all of the efflux, which also contributes to a dryer workplace. We use a funneled apron spanned between the table under the patient and the operator to catch the efflux and funnel it into a graduated receptacle.

Electronic scales to measure weight differences are more convenient than subtracting volumes but not more accurate. Both methods are subject to spillage and transtubal loss of fluid into the abdominal cavity.

Impedance cardiography, a noninvasive method of determining volume uptake, was developed in the early 1980s but did not gain wide acceptance (van Deyk et al. 1981). Another possibility of calculating the shifted volume is measuring the alcohol concentration in the expired air after adding 96% ethanol to the irrigation fluid to a volume percentage of two. The volume shift can be calculated with the Widmark formula, which is used in forensic medicine to determine blood alcohol levels (Rancke et al. 1992, Hahn & Ekengren 1993).

Rarely are more than 300 mL to 500 mL of an irrigant shifted to the systemic circulation at a maxi-

mum intrauterine pressure of 70 mmHg to 150 mmHg during the maximum of 30 minutes to 40 minutes that an operative hysteroscopic procedure usually takes. Healthy patients usually tolerate shifts of up to 1000 mL without symptoms and with only slight biochemical and hematologic changes (Molnár et al. 1992). Accordingly, monitoring fluid balance by comparing influx and efflux volumes at intervals of 5 minutes to 10 minutes provides adequate safety. The operation should be interrupted if the volume shift excedes 1000 mL or if clinical symptoms develop.

CO_2 *Hysteroscopy*

CO_2 has a permanent place in gynecological endoscopy as a medium for producing pneumoperitoneum for laparoscopy. It is an "embolism-free" gas since it is, to a great degree, dissolved in blood. Van der Pas has reported that 54.1 mL of CO_2 can be dissolved in 100 mL of blood at 37 °C without bubble formation. According to Lindemann (1976, etc.), the total gas volume necessary for CO_2 hysteroscopy is exhaled during its first passage through the lungs so that there are no changes in pH or other values measured at routine blood-gas analysis (Fig. **20**).

Special insufflators have been developed for hysteroscopy. Insufflators for laparoscopy should not be used. Larger amounts of gas, such as those introduced with pertubation apparatuses or insufflators for laparoscopy can cause mild cardiac arrhythmias as well as severe complications, such as cardiac or

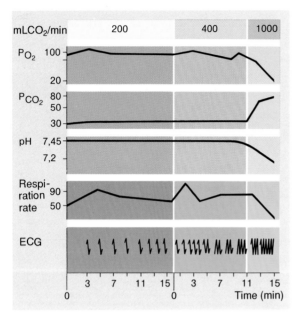

Fig. **21** Animal experiments of CO_2 hysteroscopy (Lindemann, Atlas der Hysteroskopie, Gustav Fischer Verlag 1980, Stuttgart)

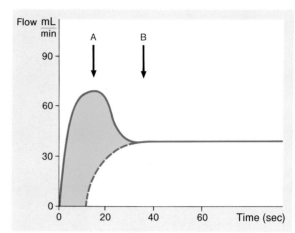

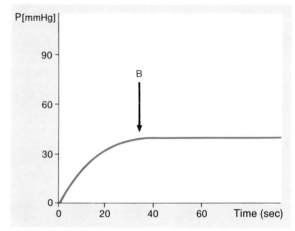

Fig. **22** Correlation between flow and time at given intracavitary pressures (Gallinat and Lücken, 1984)

pulmonary arrest. In studies on conscious dogs, Lindemann found that cardiac arrhythmias were the first sign of a too high flow of CO_2. Such signs should be recognized as warning signals during hysteroscopy (Fig. **21**). Lindemann first insufflated 200 mL/minute of CO_2 intravenously and observed that cardiac and respiratory compensatory mechanisms kept blood gases within normal limits. When the CO_2 flow was raised to 400 mL/minute, the respiration rate and then the respiratory volume increased while blood gases remained stable. Disturbances in cardiac rhythm, however, appeared relatively soon. When the flow was increased to 1000 mL/minute, after only a short time blood CO_2 increased, blood O_2 dropped, the pH rapidly shifted into acidosis, the respiration rate fell, and bundle-branch blocks appeared in the electrocardiogram.

Such complications have rarely been reported and need not be feared with modern hysteroflators. These apparatuses enable the operator either to limit the flow, by which the intrauterine pressure can be regulated continuously, or to set the intrauterine pressure not to exceed a defined value (Fig. **22**).

An intrauterine pressure of 50 to 70 mmHg usually suffices for hysteroscopy. Even under difficult conditions, we have never needed an intrauterine pressure of over 100 mmHg or a flow of more than 100 mL/minute.

In contrast to dextran solution, CO_2 is not a nuisance for the patient or the operator and makes no particular demands on the instruments. Thus, for most hysteroscopists, CO_2 insufflation has become the method of choice for distending the uterine cavity.

Fig. **23** CO$_2$ hysteroflator. This pump permits presetting of maximum gas pressure and flow

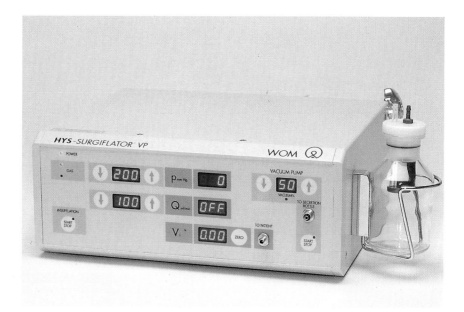

Fig. **24** Cold-light source with continuous regulation of light intensity and automatic adaptation of brightness

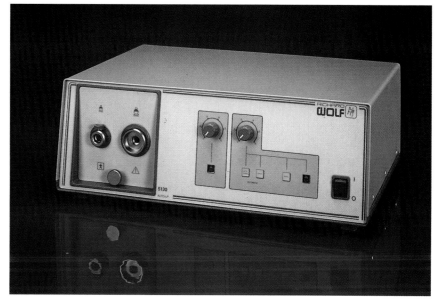

Hysteroflators

The hysteroflators currently on the market are designed especially for insufflating CO$_2$. They are equipped with a CO$_2$ cylinder or cartridge. The principle of all these devices is the same. To avoid the complications described above, the flow, the intrauterine pressure, or both are controlled. Most insufflators still contain a vacuum pump for applying a cervical adapter (Fig. 23). An manometer or digital display shows intrauterine pressure or CO$_2$ flow. The intrauterine pressure is limited to 200 mmHg and the flow to a maximum of 100 mL/minute.

The hysteroflators on the market allow preselection of the intrauterine pressure flow (Fig. **23**). Some instruments permit preselection of both pressure and flow. Some systems now have the option of attaching a printer to the hysteroflator to record gas flow and pressure versus time. Whether these curves reflect tubal patency or occlusion in the sense of tubal pertubation with CO$_2$ is under study. In any case, the operator should be able to rely on the insufflation machine to keep the intrauterine pressure and flow below the critical limits so that he or she can concentrate fully on the procedure.

Cold-light Sources

All high-energy cold-light sources with an output of over 150 watts are suitable (Fig. **24**). Less powerful light sources cannot optimally illuminate the visual field. In addition to these light sources, which are fully adequate for routine practice, special light sources and lamps have been designed for film and photo documentation.

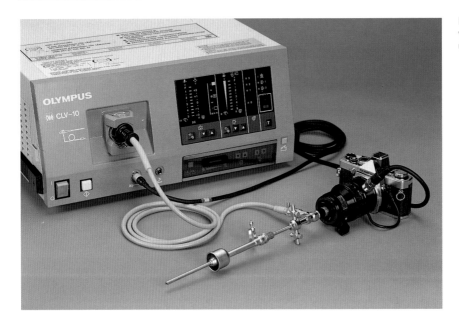

Fig. **25** Cold-light source with computer-assisted flash unit for photodocumentation

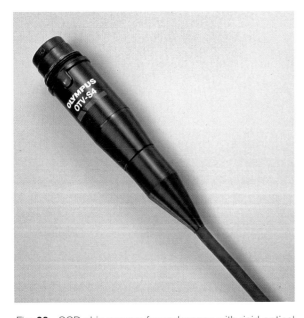

Fig. **26** CCD chip camera for endoscopy with rigid optical systems

Photographic and Video Documentation

The documentation of hysteroscopic findings on film or video serves scientific and educational purposes. Special cold-light sources have been designed for research and teaching centers. Photographic documentation requires a reflex camera that measures the light intensity at the film and sets the exposure times accordingly. Lenses with fixed or continuously adjustable focal lengths are available for endoscopic photography.

There are two possibilities for photographic documentation. Photography can be carried out under the intensive constant light from the cold-light source. This requires relatively long exposure times. The alternative is a flash system designed for endophotography (Fig. **25**). In such a system, the duration of the flash is set by computer, and correct exposure is indicated by an acoustic or visual signal. If the signal does not appear, the lens has to be moved closer to the object and a new picture taken.

Modern endocameras for video documentation contain CCD chips and weigh roughly 50 g (Fig. **26**). With these systems the entire procedure can be followed on the monitor (Fig. **27**).

At diagnostic procedures, which generally take only a few minutes, videohysteroscopy is useful for educational purposes and documentation. But during operative hysteroscopy, which can take 40 minutes, a video system is almost essential to avoid an awkward position for the operator and to permit better manipulation (Fig. **27**). It takes some practice to maintain spatial orientation during videohysteroscopy, especially during surgical procedures. Beam splitters are no longer widely used because of light loss, and operators who are unsure of their spatial orientation, and thus in danger of perforating the uterus, should not hesitate to remove the camera and orient themselves by direct vision.

Videotapes can be made with recorders that can be connected with text generators. Videoprinters can produce color or black-and-white prints during the procedure or from a videotape.

Sterilization

A sterile hysteroscope should be used for each patient.

After use, the instrument should be taken apart and cleaned. The surgical channel should be cleaned carefully from the inside to remove blood or debris before it hardens. The instrument is then disinfected in a specially designed system. Hysteroscopes can be sterilized with gas or steam or soaked in a solution. Gas sterilization is generally an option only for hospitals because such systems are usually too expensive for offices. Steam sterilization has the disadvantage that the cement in which the lenses are mounted becomes brittle with time. Recently, however, a cement has been developed that can withstand conventional steam disinfection. If gas sterilization is unavailable, if the scope may not be suitable for steam disinfection, or if the instrument is older, it is better to immerse it in a sterilizing solution and then to pack it in sterile towels. Before renewed use, the instrument should be immersed again for a short time in the solution. For gas or steam sterilization, appropriate containers are available in various sizes (Fig. 28).

Because the quality of the finish and the durability of instruments from different manufacturers can differ slightly, the disinfection and sterilization facilities at the site where it is to be used should be considered when buying a hysteroscopy system.

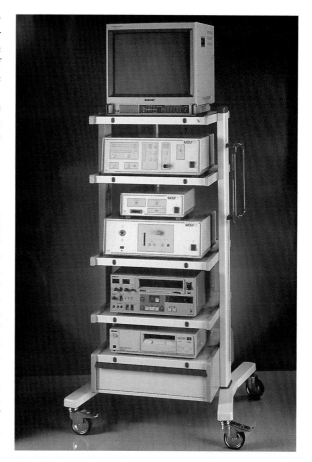

Fig. 27 Complete endoscopy tower with equipment for video recording and documentation

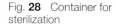

Fig. 28 Container for sterilization

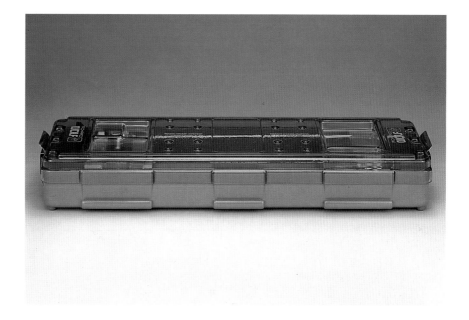

Indications for Hysteroscopy

The catalog of indications for hysteroscopy is increasing steadily. Established indications (Table 1) must be distinguished from research purposes (Table 2).

Table **1**   Established indications for hysteroscopy

Diagnostic hysteroscopy
– Abnormal uterine bleeding – Infertility and sterility – Abnormal vaginal ultrasound findings – Unclear cytologic findings – Follow-up of endometrial hyperplasia – Intrauterine staging of endometrial cancer
Operative hysteroscopy
– Extraction of a "lost" intrauterine device (IUD) – Ablation or resection of the endometrium – Resection of septa, myomas, and polyps in patients with infertility or abnormal bleeding – Lysis of adhesions in Asherman's syndrome

Table **2**   Research indications for hysteroscopy

– Chorionic biopsy – Transcervical sterilization

Abnormal Uterine Bleeding

Hysteroscopy has proved effective in the workup of patients with abnormal uterine bleeding, particularly after curettage has yielded no abnormal findings. Our experience confirms that of Lübke (1983) and Word et al. (1958), who reported that 30% to 40% of endometrial polyps were missed by currettage and then caused refractory bleeding.

Small submucosal myomas are also usually missed by curettage. Some of them can be removed hysteroscopically; some are an indication for hysterectomy.

Hysteroscopy for investigation of the endometrium can be performed on an inpatient or outpatient basis. Outpatient hysteroscopy can spare the patient a hospital stay when endoscopy shows that a fractional curettage will yield no abnormal findings. Hysteroscopy before conventional fractional dilation and curettage can identify lesions such as endometrial polyps and submucosal myomas immediately, thus allowing specific therapeutic measures. Particularly polyps in the uterine cavity can be difficult to catch and remove with the curet, even for experienced operators.

Infertility and Sterility

Uterine malformations and intrauterine adhesions or myomas can cause infertility. These conditions can be diagnosed and evaluated in detail using hysteroscopy, and further treatment can be planned.

Abnormal Vaginal Smears

Abnormal vaginal smears without a colposcopic substrate suggest a lesion of the endocervix or endometrium and are an indication for hysteroscopy. Morphologically tangible intrauterine lesions can thus be diagnosed and their extent defined. Likewise, over-interpretations that have led to a diagnosis of a grade III Papanicolaou smear can be corrected. In cases in which the lesions seems to lie in the endocervix, we have found the combination of outpatient hysteroscopy and endocervical curettage to be helpful.

Staging of Endometrial Carcinoma

Fractional curettage has been the method of choice for the diagnosis and intrauterine staging of endometrial carcinoma. However, we have seen that the endocervical fraction is contaminated by material from the uterine cavity in up to 75% of cases (thus yielding a false positive diagnosis of stage II disease according to the 1971 FIGO classification). Hysteroscopy is able to define precisely the intrauterine spread of the disease.

"Lost" Intrauterine Device

Hysteroscopy is the method of choice for removing a "lost" IUD, especially after failed attempts to retrieve the IUD blindly or under ultrasound guidance.

Endometrial Ablation and Resection of Uterine Myomas, Polyps, and Septa

Bleeding disorders such as hypermenorrhea and polymenorrhea in patients with small but diffusely myohypertrophic uteri are now treated increasingly by hysteroscopic ablation or resection of the endometrium after malignancy has been ruled out. Submucous myomas or polyps protruding into the uterine cavity and causing bleeding disorders or infertility can also be resected hysteroscopically. High-frequency resecto-scopes and electrodes used in a fluid distension medium are widely preferred to the Nd:YAG laser with a bare fiber. All patients should receive a progestin, GnRH analogue, or danazol for 2 months to 3 months before the procedure. Synechiae and uterine mal-formations such as septa, which can be encountered during workups for sterility and infertility, are also treated in this fashion.

Contraindications

Acute endomyometritis or salpingo-oophoritis is an absolute contraindication for hysteroscopy. An examination in a patient with acute pelvic inflammatory disease (PID) can exacerbate the condition. Chronic PID is only a relative contraindication. Reviewing 4000 hysteroscopies, Salat-Baroux et al. (1984) found only seven cases of subsequent PID. These cases may have been caused by the procedure itself, or they may have been exacerbations of chronic conditions. In 1100 hysteroscopies, we have seen only one case of acute PID that may have been provoked by the procedure. This was a premenopausal patient with dysfunctional bleeding who had reported recurring episodes of PID in her medical history. At the time of hysteroscopy she was free of complaints, and the gynecologic examination was normal; two days later she was admitted to the hospital with acute PID. These complications support Siegler's theory that the endometrium has a special, but as yet unclear, defense mechanism (Siegler, personal communication, 1992).

Exacerbation of chronic, recurrent PID is an infrequent but typical complication of hysteroscopy. In patients with a history of recurrent PID or in those with suggestive findings at palpation, a leukocyte count and erythrocyte sedimentation rate should be obtained before hysteroscopy. These examinations are not necessary if there is no clinical or medical history of PID.

Profuse uterine bleeding is a relative contraindication to hysteroscopy because the bleeding usually is so severe that an exact diagnosis is impossible. Also, hysteroscopy generally should not be performed during the second half of the menstrual cycle, particularly in patients being treated for sterility. The possibility that hysteroscopy disturbs implantation or tubal transport has not been ruled out. Also, in the secretory phase, the endometrium is built up, and intrauterine causes of sterility are thus much harder to recognize than in the early proliferative phase when the uterine cavity is lined only by a thin mucous membrane.

An intact intrauterine pregnancy is a further relative contraindication. Apart from the retrieval of a lost IUD in early pregnancy or chorionic biopsy, there are no indications for hysteroscopy during pregnancy (Table 3).

Table **3**   Contraindications for hysteroscopy

Absolute	– Pelvic inflammatory disease (PID) – Colpitis
Relative	– Pregnancy – Secretory phase of the menstrual cycle – Profuse uterine bleeding – Chronic PID

Complications and Side Effects

Hysteroscopy has a low rate of complications, and serious complications are rare (Table **4**). Complications can be classified as immediate or late.

Immediate Complications

Uterine Perforation

Perforation of the uterus at diagnostic hysteroscopy can almost always be avoided if careful bimanual palpation and sounding of the uterus, cervical canal, and uterine cavity are done before hysteroscopy. The narrowest point during a hysteroscopic examination is always the internal os. But when orthograde optics are used, the internal os is passed under visual control and perforation of the posterior wall or fundus of the uterus would be expected to be much less frequent than during conventional dilation and curettage. Problems can arise if the cervical canal is obliterated and has to be dilated before hysteroscopy, particularly in patients with atrophic uteri. Such perforations occur during dilation of the internal os, not during hysteroscopy.

We have not seen a perforation during outpatient hysteroscopy. Lindemann (1975, 1980, etc.) reported six perforations in a total of 5220 hysteroscopies, an incidence of about one per 1000 procedures.

CO_2 Insufflation

Today CO_2 is the medium most widely used to dilate the uterine cavity. In the late 1970s, there were reports of cardiac and respiratory arrests caused exclusively by insufflated CO_2 being absorbed into the blood stream and causing shifts in the acid–base equilibrium and gas emboli. The gas pressure was not controlled in any of these cases (Siegler 1983). In animal experiments and clinical studies, Lindemann (1975), Semm & Rimkus (1974), and Salat-Baroux et al. (1984) showed that the hysteroscopy insufflators available today have little or no influence on blood gases and the condition of the patient. In all the reported cases of fatal complications, the CO_2 flow was either well over 350 mL/minute, or the gas pressure was not monitored.

A maximum CO_2 flow of 100 mL/minute and a maximum gas pressure of 200 mm Hg are today considered sufficient to develop pneumometra. The complications discussed above were no longer seen after these guidelines were adopted (Lindemann 1988). Isolated reports of gas embolism have appeared only recently, and these were attributed to the nitrous oxide (N_2O) used for anesthesia at hysteroscopy. N_2O reduces the blood's binding capacity for CO_2 (Crozier et al. 1991). Such reports of potentially fatal complications have to be taken seriously but the question arises why a technique that has been used in thousands of patients with no complications led to severe complications in three of only 62 patients at one center. We have had no case of CO_2 embolism in our experience of over 2000 outpatient hysteroscopies.

In our experience gas pressures of 30 mmHg to 70 mmHg generally suffice to produce and maintain pneumometra. Abnormal anatomical conditions can sometimes necessitate a higher CO_2 pressure, for instance in patients with uterine leiomyomas. In such situations, the pressure is set to a higher value by the operator.

Table **4**   Complications of diagnostic hysteroscopy

Complication	Incidence	Cause	Reference
Uterine perforation	1/1000	False route	Lindemann 1980; Siegler 1983
PID	2/1000	Primary infection or exacerbation of existing infection	Hepp 1979; Salat-Baroux 1984 et al.
Pulmonary or cardiac arrest	Isolated cases	Too high CO_2 pressure	Lindemann 1975; Siegler 1983
Circulatory dysregulation	Isolated cases	Reaction to local anesthetic	Lindemann 1980
Tumor cell spread	Conceivable, but not proven	Intracavity pressure in excess of the tubal perturbation threshold	Neis (see p. 23)

Siegler (1983) observed the rupture of a hydrosal-pinx during a simultaneous hysteroscopy and laparas-copy. This was a rare immediate complication that required no therapy and that probably would have been noted only as a painful event during a conventional hysteroscopy. Such reports strengthen our conviction that the intracavitary pressure should be kept below 60 mmHg if at all possible. If the patient perceives pain in the area of the adnexa, this possibility must be con-sidered, and the procedure may have to be terminated prematurely.

Distension with Liquid Media

Liquid distension media can be absorbed into the systemic circulation through the wound surface of the operative field. The extent of such fluid shifts depends on the nature of the procedure, its duration, and the intrauterine pressure (see "Continuous-Flow Hystero-scopy"). The result is hypotonic hyperhydration with hyponatremia (fluid overload and water intoxication). Clinical symptoms include a sudden blood pressure increase with bradycardia and circulatory depression; neurologic symptoms; oliguria, anuria or acute renal failure; and pulmonary edema (Greene 1982, Harz-mann & van Deyk 1982, Zwergel 1987, Witz et al. 1993). The fluid-overload syndrome, known in urology as the "post-TURP syndrome," is potentially fatal but usually not seen in healthy patients if the shifted volume is less than 1000 mL (Molnár et al. 1992). Because the shifted volumes at operative hysteroscopy are usually less than 1000 mL (Magos et al. 1989), the fluid-overload syndrome is usually not a problem if fluid is balanced meticulously during surgery. In a review of 2796 endometrial ablations, Macdonald et al. (1992) reported a 0.3 % incidence of the fluid-overload syndrome.

Other side effects of fluid distension media depend on the medium itself (see also "Liquid Distension Media"). Dextrans of low or intermediate molecular weight entail a risk of anaphylactic reactions, coagula-tion disorders, pulmonary edema, and respiratory distress syndrome. Solutions containing glucose can cause hyperglycemia. Solutions containing glycine seem to entail an increased risk of fluid overload and severe neurotoxic side effects due to the metabolic product, ammonia. Semi-iso-osmolar solutions of mannitol and sorbitol should be used only in patients with normal liver function and without fructose intolerance. Rarely, lactic acidosis can develop if large volumes are shifted. Long urologic experience suggests that media with 1.5% glycine or a combination of 0.54% mannitol and 2.7% sorbitol can be recommended.

Complications at Operative Hysteroscopy

Perforation of the uterus is the most common compli-cation at hysteroscopic myomectomy, endometrial ablation, or septum resection and occurs in 1% to 2%

of procedures (Macdonald et al. 1991, Magos et al. 1991). Perforation is usually mechanical. The idea that some of the lesions are due to thermal energy and secondary necrosis is contradicted by laparoscopic measurements of temperature at the serosal surface of the uterus during intracavitary high-frequency electro-surgery. At a power setting of 50 watts and 150 watts for dissection and coagulation, the temperature increase at the serosa was less than 6 °C (Indman & Brown 1992).

Endomyometritis is about half as common as perforation. Complications requiring laparotomy, such as lesions of the bowel, bladder, ureter, or major vessels (Lindemann 1980, Siegler 1984) occur at an incidence of up to 1 per 1000 procedures. The incidence of severe postoperative bleeding or sepsis is similar. Notably, uterine perforation is most common during a surgeon's first five resectoscopic procedures, and severe injuries, such as those involving the bowel, are more likely if the operation is not supervised by an experienced colleague (Macdonald et al. 1991).

All in all, the risks associated with operative hysteroscopy are low if the procedure is performed or supervised by an experienced operator. Conventional hysterectomy, often the alternative avoided by opera-tive hysteroscopy, entails a surgical mortality rate of 0.06% to 0.16% and a rate of severe complications of 1.0% to 2.5% (Dicker et al. 1982, Wingo et al. 1983, Loft et al. 1991).

Complications Associated with Anesthesia

If hysteroscopy is performed during intubation or mask anesthesia before a fractional curettage, the insufflated CO_2 will be exhaled during its first pass through the lungs before it affects blood-gas concentrations. Because of reports of gas emboli associated with the use of nitrous oxide (Crozier et al. 1991) (see p. 21), this gas should not be used for general anesthesia for hysteroscopy, which is usually of short duration. Early signs of intraoperative gas embolism are a drop in the CO_2 concentration of the expired air and increased CO_2 in the peripheral blood. A cogwheel murmur ausculta-ted over the heart signals the transition from laminar to turbulent blood flow. Transesophageal or precardiac Doppler ultrasonography are more sensitive in detec-ting CO_2 bubbles in the circulation.

Modern standard 4-mm hysteroscopes can usually be used without general anesthesia. A paracervical block is sometimes necessary, and local anesthetic agents can lead to circulatory dysregulation and methemoglobin formation. Lindemann's group (1980) has reported seeing no more such side effects since they began using articaine hydrochloride.

Allergic reactions to local anesthetic agents have not been reported during hysteroscopy but the patient should be asked about a history of any such reactions.

During operative hysteroscopy with a fluid disten-sion medium, the symptoms of fluid overload and water intoxication should be watched for closely. If a patient receiving regional anesthesia reports headaches or shows confusion, the operation should be stopped immediately and anesthesiologic countermeasures (administration of sodium, diuretics, and glucocorticoids) should be taken.

Late Complications

Infections

The rate of infectious complications after hysteroscopy lies between 0.5% and 2%. This is assuming that the relative and absolute contraindications discussed above are observed.

Dissemination of Tumor Cells

Studies by the Gynecologic Oncology Group (GOG) have shown a surprisingly high rate of tumor cells in the peritoneal cavity in patients with endometrial cancer. In a total of 747 patients, the cytology of fluid from peritoneal lavages was positive in 7.7% of those with stage I disease and 21% of those with stage II disease (DiSaia 1982).

This raises the issue of whether applying positive pressure in the uterine cavity can push tumor cells into the abdomen. Johnson (1973) and Joelsson et al. (1971) followed up a total of more than 700 patients 5-14 years after hysterography. The survival time and the recurrence rate were unchanged. Joelsson even found that passage of contrast medium into the tubes was a favorable prognostic sign. Possibly, the tubal ostia are occluded by tumor more often in advanced stages of disease than in early stages.

The issue of tumor cell spread during hysteroscopy has received only scant study (Nagel et al. 1984), particularly with the use of CO_2 as the dilation medium

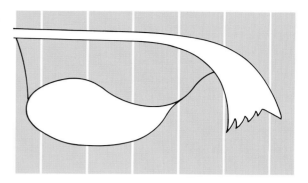

Fig. **29**   Schematic representation of the sectioning of the uterine adnexa (Department of Obstetrics and Gynecology, University of Hamburg)

(Cittadini et al. 1985). We have performed hysteroscopy in a total of 94 patients with endometrial carcinoma. Seventy-two of these patients subsequently underwent surgery appropriate for the disease stage, two patients in poor medical condition underwent only vaginal hysterectomy, and 20 women received radiotherapy (Table 5). Thus, the tubes of 73 patients were available for histology. Since the adnexa of patients with a uterine malignancy are embedded in toto at our pathology laboratory, these tubes could be completely reassessed. The sectioning of the adnexa is shown in Figs. **29** and **30.** The adnexa are embedded in five to eight fractions, according to size. For this study, three

Table **5**   Treatment of 94 patients with endometrial carcinoma who underwent hysteroscopy

Surgery appropriate for stage	72
Vaginal hysterectomy	2
Radiation therapy	20
Total	94

Fig. **30** Sectioned and fixated adnexa

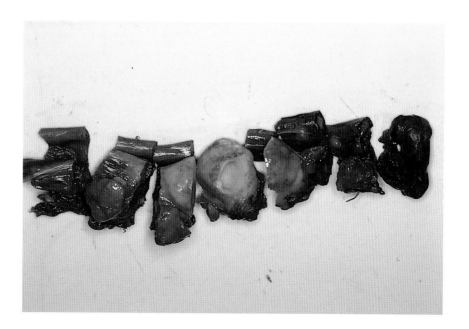

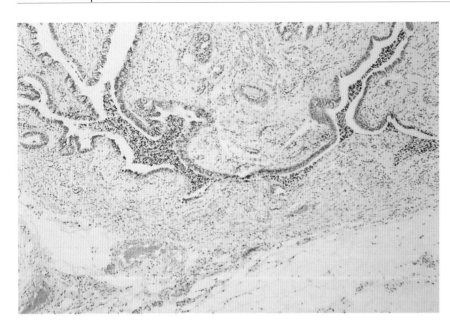

Fig. **31**   Histologic picture of a tubal section. The lumen contains degenerated tubal epithelium but no tumor cells. HE stain, X 30

step-serial sections were obtained per fraction so that 15 to 24 slices were available for each tube.

Viable tumor cells were not found in any of the tubes. In 6 patients, isolated deposits of necrotic tissue were found in the tubal lumina. It could not be ruled out with certainty that these deposits stemmed from the uterine cavity, but they probably were necrotic tubal villi (Fig. **31**). Lymphangiosis carcinomatosa of the right mesovarium was found in one patient.

These morphological results were then compared with the patients' clinical courses. Since we began performing hysteroscopy in endometrial cancer patients in 1981, only the 2-year recurrence-free rate and the 2-year survival rate based on 73 women are available; 55 of these patients underwent surgery and 16 received radiotherapy (Table **6**).

Table **6**   Outcome of 73 patients with endometrial carcinoma who underwent hysteroscopy and were followed up for more than 2 years

Died of recurrence	4
Survived intrauterine recurrence	2
Died of other causes	3
2-year survival rate	91.4 %
Adjusted 2-year survival rate	95 %

Four patients died of tumor recurrence; two patients with intrauterine recurrence after primary radiotherapy underwent secondary surgery and were free of disease thereafter; and three patients died of cardiovascular disease.

The 2-year survival rate of our patients is 91.4% (corrected, 95%) and thus no lower than the average of the values in the FIGO *Annual Report of the Results of Treatment of Gynecological Cancer* (Kottmeier 1985).

All four of the women who died of recurrence within the first 2 years had undifferentiated carcinomas (Table 7).

Table **7**   Data of four patients who died of recurrent endometrial carcinoma after prior hysteroscopy

Patient	FIGO stage	Depth of myometrial invasion	Grading	Other
1	IV	Unknown	3	Vaginal and lung metastases
2	I	3/3	3	–
3	III	3/3	3	–
4	I	Unknown	3	Incomplete radiation therapy

The two patients who had undergone surgery had myometrial invasion almost to the serosa. In the two patients treated with radiation, therapy was interrupted in one because of poor general condition and advanced age and in the other because of distant metastases at the time of diagnosis.

This review and other published reports show no detrimental effects of hysteroscopy on the course of patients with endometrial cancer. This appraisal is based on the following observations:

1. Careful processing and microscopic inspection of the tubes of patients who underwent surgery showed no viable tumor cells in any of the tubal lumens.
2. The 2-year survival rate did not differ from that reported in the literature.

3. All patients who died during follow-up had poor prognoses to begin with.

We thus think that hysteroscopy is neither absolutely nor relatively contraindicated in patients with endometrial carcinoma. There is no indication in the literature that hysteroscopy or hysterography has an adverse effect on the course of the disease. The GOG data (DiSaia et al. 1983) suggest that tumor cells found by peritoneal lavage rarely if ever develop into metastases; if the opposite were true, peritoneal carcinomatosis would be seen much more frequently in patients with endometrial cancer. Also, Creasman & Lukeman (1972) reported finding tumor cells of endometrial carcinoma in the abdominal cavity in patients with ligated or missing tubes.

Side Effects

Side effects of hysteroscopy are seen almost only in procedures perfomed without analgesia or paracervical block. Occasionally, pain can be caused by irritation of the peritoneum and phrenic nerve by CO_2 (Lindemann 1980). Shoulder pain occurred during our early hysteroscopies, which took considerably more time than the average of 2 minutes that they do now. After reducing intrauterine pressure, we now hear such complaints very rarely.

La Sala et al. (1984) reported on lower abdominal pain similar to menstrual cramps during or after hysteroscopy. These cramps probably are a result of contractions of the uterine musculature trying to counter the dilation. They are seen almost only in premenopausal women, particularly in those with a history of dysmenorrhea.

We have had only two patients with cramping pain after hysteroscopy severe enough to require medication. The pain resolved completely after 15 minutes in one patient and 1 hour in the other.

We have seen circulatory disturbances, particularly during our early procedures. These occurred almost exclusively in patients who were anxious and tense during the entire examination and who then, after sitting up, complained of dizziness and nausea. In such cases, we ask the patient to lie back down and reassure her. The symptoms disappear within 5 to 10 minutes; no patient has had to be admitted to the hospital.

Examination Procedure

A medical history should be taken and the indication for hysteroscopy reviewed before the procedure. To avoid complications, the relative and absolute contraindications should be observed (Table **8**).

The patient is placed in the dorsal lithotomy position. Premedication is not necessary for outpatient procedures. A bimanual gynecologic examination is performed to determine the position of the uterus and its relation to the neighboring organs. The vagina is then opened with a duck-billed speculum, and the cervix and vagina are disinfected with an appropriate solution. Next, a tenaculum is applied to the cervix at 12 o'clock. We have found it helpful to ask the patient to cough when applying the tenaculum. Local anesthesia, for example with ethyl chloride, produces no better effect. The uterine cavity is then sounded with a 3-mm probe to determine the axis of the cervical canal and uterine cavity and the size of the uterus. If, during an outpatient examination, the patient reports pain when the internal os is passed with the 3-mm probe, a paracervical block should be considered.

Hysteroscopy itself begins with introducing the optical system into the cervical canal (Fig. **32**). The uterus is extended by pulling on the tenaculum, and the hysteroscope is advanced under visual control to the internal os.

Table **8**   Procedure for diagnostic hysteroscopy

Absolute contraindication	Relative contraindication	No contraindication
Acute endomyometritis	Pregnancy	Gynecologic examination ↓
Salpingo-oophoritis	Second half of the menstrual cycle	Insertion of the duck-billed speculum ↓
Colpitis	Heavy uterine bleeding	Disinfection of the vagina ↓
Specific therapy before hysteroscopy	Chronic PID	Application of a tenaculum to the cervix at 12 o'clock ↓
	Check WBC and ESR before hysteroscopy	Sounding the cervical canal (local anesthesia?) ↓
		Is dilation necessary? ↓
		Hysteroscopy

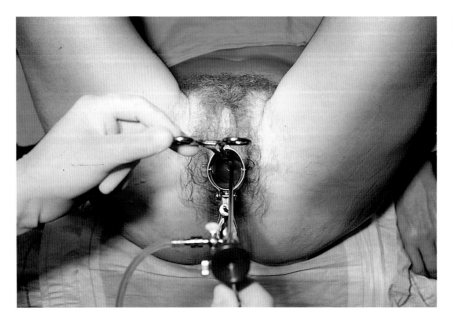

Fig. **32**   Introduction of the hysteroscope into the cervical canal after application of a tenaculum to the cervix at 12 o'clock

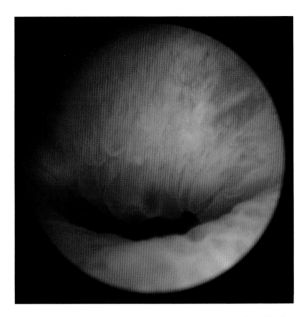

Fig. **33** View into the cervical canal during slow insufflation of CO_2

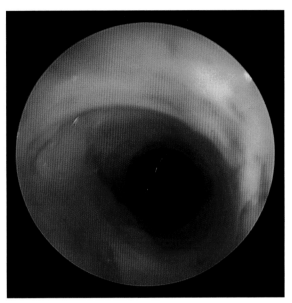

Fig. **34** The cervical canal is completely unfolded

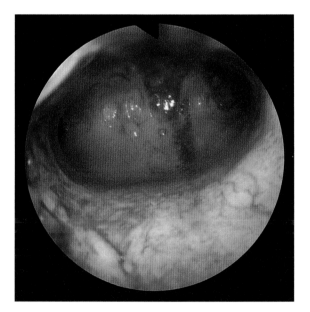

Fig. **35** View from the uterine isthmus into the uterine cavity

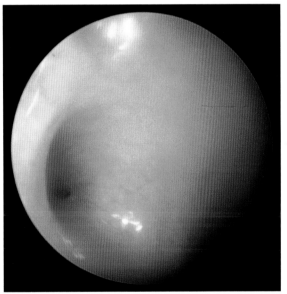

Fig. **36** The right tubal ostium

A steady stream of CO_2 opens the cervical canal in front of the scope (Figs. **33, 34**). CO_2 also enters the uterine cavity, which can be surveyed as soon as the scope passes the internal os (Fig. **35**).

The uterine cavity should be inspected in a systematic manner. We prefer the following procedure:

1. Inspection of the cervical canal
2. Panoramic survey of the uterine cavity
3. Inspection of the uterine fundus
4. Inspection of the right and left tubal angles (Fig. **36**)

5. Inspection of the anterior, posterior, and right and left walls of the uterine cavity (Figs. **37, 38**)

Attention is paid to anatomical features such as uterine malformations and submucosal leiomyomas jutting into the lumen of the uterus and to distortion of the cavity by intramural leiomyomas. The endometrium is evaluated, and any lesions are assessed for malignancy. Samples of the endometrium are obtained for cytology and histology (see "Morphological Confirmation of Endoscopic Findings").

During hysteroscopy pneumometra is maintained by the hysteroflator. If possible, the intracavity

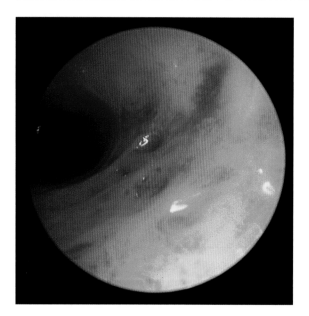

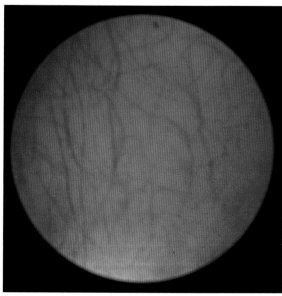

Fig. **37** Inspection of the lateral walls of the uterine cavity

Fig. **38** Fine vascular pattern of normal endometrium, recognizable with the end of the hysteroscope in contact with the mucous membrane

pressure should be kept below the tubal pertubation threshold of 60 mmHg. If this pressure does not produce pneumometra, the intracavity pressure can be raised accordingly. We have never needed a pressure of more than 100 mmHg or a flow of more than 100 mL/minute.

The cold-light source is a 250-watt halogen lamp that has a flash generator with a maximum of 600 watts. Photographic documentation is performed with a reflex camera with a zoom lens. We have found a printed form useful to document the findings of the examination. It contains the relevant data from the medical history, the indication for the procedure, the optics used, the course of the examination, the findings, and any complications (Fig. **39**). The form is designed so that it can be used to formulate a medical report. Finally, the hysteroscopic diagnosis and the histologic results are used to plan further therapy.

UNIVERSITÄTS-FRAUENKLINIK u.
POLIKLINIK
6650 HOMBURG (SAAR)

Hysteroscopy Report

Date ☐☐☐☐☐

Patient identification

Age ☐☐   Last menstrual period ☐☐☐☐☐

Vaginal deliveries ☐☐   Cycle ....

Spontaneous abortions ☐☐   Menopause .... YRS

Previous D & C/Uterine Surgery ....

Hormone therapy/Oral contraceptives ....

Day of cycle   Pap   Obesity yes ☐ no ☐

Indications/Clinical symptoms

Operative hysteroscope ☐   Contact microcolpohysteroscope ☐   Minihysteroscope ☐

Analgesia   Passage of the internal os

None ☐   Easy ☐   Uterine cavity (cm) ....   Streak curette ☐
General anesthesia ☐   Difficult ☐   Dilation ....   Endometrial cytology ☐
Spinal anesthesia ☐   Impossible ☐   Fractional curettage ☐
Paracervical block ☐   Photodocumtentation ☐
Other ☐

Anterior wall   Posterior wall   Lateral walls
rt   lt   rt   lt   rt   lt
Fundus   Cervix

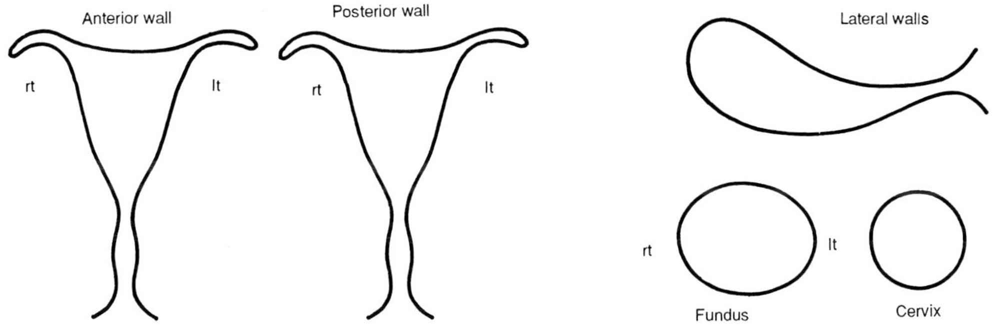

Hysteroscopy findings

Cervical canal: ....   Cavity: ....
Isthmus: ....
Endometrium: ....
Relief: ....   Rt ostium: ....
Color: ....   Lt ostium: ....
Complications: ....
Assessment:

Diagnosis:

Recommendation:

Signature

Fig. **39** Hysteroscopy report form

Hysteroscopy with or without Anesthesia?

Whether hysteroscopy will be performed with or without anesthesia essentially depends on local conditions. Outpatient hysteroscopy is carried out primarily in private gynecologic offices and in hospitals with outpatient clinics. If hysteroscopy is performed in a patient referred for inpatient fractional curettage, both procedures are carried out under general anesthesia.

In most patients being treated for sterility, laparoscopy is performed if noninvasive methods have failed. Because this procedure is performed with general anesthesia, hysteroscopy should be carried out at the same time. Hysteroscopy is no further burden for the patient, and it can yield findings relevant for further management (see "Investigation of Sterility and Infertility").

A further indication for hysteroscopy during general anesthesia is menometrorrhagia in patients with uterine leiomyomas before hysterectomy. Even if endometrial carcinoma is considered unlikely, it should nonetheless be ruled out by hysteroscopy directly before hysterectomy. This obviates the need for prior fractional curettage and the ensuing delay while waiting for the histology results, and it avoids a surprise diagnosis from histopathology of the surgical specimen (Lübke 1984).

All hysteroscopic operations should be carried out with general or spinal anesthesia because even the removal of polyps is painful.

Outpatient Hysteroscopy

Outpatient hysteroscopy is performed almost exclusively for diagnostic purposes using a hysteroscope with a shaft diameter of 5 mm or less. Specific patient preparation is unnecessary. The patient leaves the office or outpatient clinic after the procedure and does not need extended recuperation. We recommend only that she be accompanied by someone to drive her home.

Instruments for Outpatient Hysteroscopy

A duck-billed speculum has proven useful for unfolding the vagina and exposing the external os. These self-holding specula have the advantage that the hysteroscopist's hands are free.

The nurse prepares a sterile bowl with 500 mL of 0.5% chlorhexidine gluconate solution or another appropriate disinfectant. A long clamp, a tenaculum, and a uterine probe lie in the solution. After the examination, these instruments are packed away as a set and sterilized (Fig. **40**). Sterile swabs soaked in the disinfectant are used to disinfect the vagina; dry swabs are used to absorb the fluid in the posterior vault of the vagina.

Acceptance

Whether a method can establish itself in clinical practice depends on the information it can yield and on how well it is tolerated by the patient. The latter is particularly important for outpatient methods.

Early hysteroscopes had large diameters, and outpatient examination was possible only with paracervical block. This is no longer necessary because modern instruments have 5-mm diameters that roughly correspond to that of the cervical canal. Apart from individual variation, the most common problem area is the internal os, an hourglass-shaped narrowing between the endocervix and the uterine cavity (Fig. **41**).

To evaluate the influence of the shaft diameter on patient acceptance of hysteroscopy, we prospectively studied 448 examinations with a 5 x 5 mm shaft, 123 with a 3.7 x 5 mm shaft, and 100 with a 4 x 4 mm shaft.

If the patient reported no pain during the instrument's passage through the internal os, passage was considered "easy." Passage was considered "difficult" if pressure had to be applied to overcome resistance at the internal os or if the patient reported pain. Some of these patients required a paracervical block. If the

Fig. **40** Instrumentarium for outpatient hysteroscopy

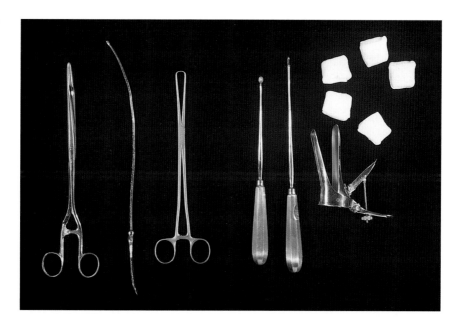

internal os could not be traversed at all, whether because of pain or anatomical reasons (e. g., steep anteflexion of the uterus, extensive leiomyomas, stenosis of the fornix, or total obliteration of the cervical canal), the procedure was considered "impossible." This group also contained the patients who were so sensitive to pain, anxious, or tense that the examination was stopped prematurely.

Acceptance of 5-mm Hysteroscopes

A standard hysteroscope with a shaft diameter of 5 x 5 mm and an optical system with a diameter of 4 mm were used. Passage of the internal os was easy in 75% of the patients, difficult in 19.2%, and impossible in 5.8%. Among the latter 26 patients, the investigation was discontinued for anatomical reasons (n = 14) or lack of patient cooperation (n = 12) (Table 9).

Table 9   Passage of the internal os with the 5-mm hysteroscope (n = 448)

Easy	336	75.0 %
Difficult	86	19.2 %
Impossible	26	5.8 %
	448	100.0 %

Paracervical block was necessary in 74 patients (16.5%). Twenty-two patients (4.9%) required dilation of the cervical canal because the scope could not be passed even after cervical blockade (Table 10). In these cases the cervical canal was dilated up to Hegar 4.5 or, at most, Hegar 5, so that gas would not escape beside the scope during the subsequent procedure.

Table 10   Additional procedures during outpatient hysteroscopy (5-mm scope) in 448 patients

Paracervical block	74	16.5 %
Dilation of the cervical canal	22	4.9 %

Other Factors

Menopausal Status

The ease of hysteroscopy differs somewhat according to age, particularly between postmenopausal patients with afunctional uteri and premenopausal patients with regular cycles and the corresponding physiological changes of the endocervix (Table 11).

Table 11   Hysteroscopic passage of the internal os according to menopausal status (n = 448)

	Easy	Difficult	Impossible
Premenopausal (n = 191)	79.9 %	16.8 %	3.3 %
Perimenopausal (n = 67)	71.6 %	22.4 %	6.0 %
Postmenopausal (n = 190)	71.8 %	20.3 %	7.9 %

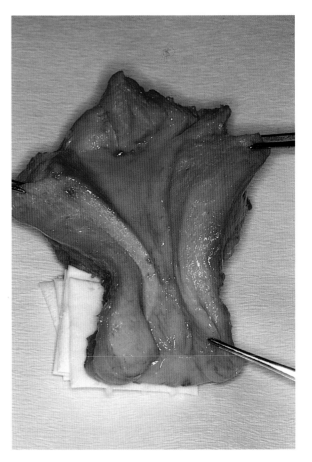

Fig. 41   Hysterectomy specimen in which the hourglass-shaped narrowing in the area of the isthmus is clearly recognizable

Access to the uterine cavity is generally easier in premenopausal women; in this age group, the rate of "impossible" hysteroscopies was 3.3% compared to 6.0% and 7.9% in perimenopausal and postmenopausal women. However, the differences among the three groups are small and not of clinical relevance.

Day of the Cycle

The patency of the cervical canal varies during the menstrual cycle. The last days of the menstrual period are best for inserting an IUD, and the middle of the cycle is best for colposcopic inspection of the squamocolumnar junction. Thus, it is to be expected that patient tolerance of hysteroscopy will vary according to the condition of the cervical canal.

We analyzed the ease of hysteroscopy in 5-day segments of the cycle in 191 patients with regular periods (Table 12). The cervix was most easily traversed from days 1 to 5 and days 10 to 20. Passage was always possible until day 5 and between days 25 and 28. Entering the uterine cavity was most difficult between days 6 and 10; the procedure was difficult in almost 30% of the patients during this phase.

Table **12**   Passage of the internal os with the 5-mm hysteroscope in 191 premenopausal patients with regular menstrual
cycles according to the day of the cycle

| Passage (%) | Day of the cycle | | | | | | |
	1-5	6-10	11-15	16-20	21-25	26-28	Average
Easy	93.3	68.2	91.3	91.7	75.8	76.5	82.2
Difficult	6.7	29.5	6.5	5.6	21.2	23.5	15.7
Impossible	0.0	2.3	2.2	2.7	3.0	0.0	2.1

Similarly, the rate of paracervical blocks was
lowest until day 5 and between days 11 and 20 (5.6%
and 6.5%, respectively, compared to an overall rate of
17.3%), and only 1 of 97 patients required dilation of
the internal os.

Thus, in more than 90 % of patients with regular
menstrual cycles, the cervical canal can be passed
easily shortly after cessation of menstrual bleeding
until day 5 of the cycle as well as between days 10 and
20. During these phases, only 6% of our patients required a paracervical block, and only 1% required
dilation of the cervical canal.

Parity

Vaginal deliveries or abortions almost always cause
recognizable changes in the cervix. The external os
resembles a dimple in nulliparas and a transverse,
sometimes gaping slot in multiparas. One would
expect hysteroscopic passage of the internal os to be
easier in multiparas than in nulliparas, and this was
confirmed in our series. The percentage of patients in
whom passage of the cervical canal was considered
easy increased from 63.2% in nulliparas to 84.9% in
women with three deliveries. Correspondingly, the
percentage of difficult or impossible examinations
decreased from 26.3% to 13.7% and from 10.5% to
1.4%, respectively (Table **13**).

Table **13**   Passage of the cervical canal with a 5-mm hysteroscope according to parity

| Passage (%) | Parity | | | | | |
	0	1	2	3	4	Average
Easy	63.2	76.9	78.6	84.9	75.5	75.8
Difficult	26.3	17.6	15.4	13.7	22.6	19.1
Impossible	10.5	5.5	6.0	1.4	1.9	5.1

Surprisingly, hysteroscopy was difficult in 22.6%
of women with four or more deliveries, a percentage
almost as high as that in nulliparas. The same holds true
for the rate of paracervical blocks and dilation. The
reason for this is unclear, but the differences may disappear when larger numbers of patients are analyzed.

Prior Operations on the Cervix

Prior surgical procedures on the cervix would be
expected to influence the ease of passage of the

hysteroscope through the internal os. Scarring from a
conization would be expected to impede hysteroscopy. Dilation and curettage might either cause
scarring or leave the cervical canal permanently
somewhat wider. In practice, we have found post-
conization scarring to complicate hysteroscopy.
Passage of the cervical canal was easy in only 46% of
13 such patients, the smallest percentage in all analyzed subgroups. In contrast, prior dilation and curettage had no effect (Table **14**).

Table **14**   Influence of prior cervical operations on the
passage of the 5-mm hysteroscope through the cervical
canal in a total of 448 patients

| Passage (%) | Prior Cervical Operation | | |
	None (n = 297)	Currettage (n = 138)	Conization (n = 13)
Easy	75.8	76.1	46.2
Difficult	18.1	19.6	38.5
Impossible	6.1	4.3	15.3

Acceptance of Hysteroscopes Measuring 3.7 x 5 mm and 4 x 4 mm

In addition to the standard 4-mm optics with a shaft
measuring 5 x 5 mm, 3-mm optics with a shaft measuring either 3.7 x 5 mm or 4 x 4 mm are available. The
field of view of the 3-mm optical system is much
narrower than that of the 4-mm system, and the light
intensity is much weaker. Both a survey of the uterine
cavity and inspection of details is difficult. Satisfactory
photographic documentation is very difficult.

We have used hysteroscopes measuring 3.7 x
5 mm and 4 x 4 mm in 123 and 100 consecutive
patients, respectively, under the same conditions as the
4-mm optical systems. The patients did not differ with
respect to age distribution, menopausal status, parity,
or indications for hysteroscopy.

We found that in women with very narrow cervical canals, usually nulliparas, the thin hysteroscopes
could be used without anesthesia and thus had a certain
advantage over the 5-mm scope. However, in 20% of
the overall collective, CO_2 escaped through the cervical canal around the narrow hysteroscopes, thus
preventing satisfactory pneumometra.

Since the optical quality of these small hysteroscopes is inferior, it is unlikely that they will establish
themselves for routine diagnostics. They are instruments for specific situations and round out the
instrumentarium of hysteroscopists who perform large
numbers of procedures.

Optimal Timing of Examination

Overall, outpatient hysteroscopy with standard 5-mm
instruments is unproblematic in about 80% of patients
and painful in about 20%. This 20% is made up of
patients in whom the internal os can be passed after

dilation (15%) and those in whom the procedure is impossible (5%).

Filshie and Nicolaides (1983) reported using synthetic laminary stents to dilate the cervical canal. Other groups have used locally applied prostaglandins (Rath 1985; Hald et al. 1988). Both these modalities have the disadvantage that they must be applied up to 24 hours before hysteroscopy. Also, both the swelling of the laminary stents and prostaglandin-induced uterine contractions can cause lower abdominal pain. Laminary stents can cause uterine infections and local application of prostaglandins occasionally causes systemic side effects (Hald et al. 1988).

In our experience, local application of prostaglandins can widen the cervical canal to the extent that the internal os does not fit snugly around the instrument, thus allowing gas to escape and preventing effective pneumometra.

In premenopausal women, hysteroscopy during the second half of the cycle is relatively contraindicated since an early pregnancy could be disturbed. The second half of the cycle is appropriate only study the endometrium in patients with bleeding disorders. For other indications, particularly investigation of sterility and infertility, hysteroscopy should be carried out directly after cessation of menstrual bleeding. At this time, passage through the uterine cervix is relatively easy, and the thin endometrium does not obscure details of the uterine cavity.

In perimenopausal and postmenopausal patients there are obviously no considerations as to the day of the menstrual cycle.

Paracervical Block

If analgesia is required for hysteroscopy, a paracervical block is the technique of choice. To avoid unnecessary patient discomfort, it should be administered if the patient reports pain when the uterine sound is passed through the internal os before hysteroscopy itself. The technique is simple and does not take much time. The complication rate is low. No preparation is necessary, and the procedure is limited to those patients who report discomfort during preliminary examination.

Technique

Adequate analgesia is usually achieved by injecting 5 mL of a local anesthetic agent into each sacrouterine ligament. The effect is immediate so that sounding of the internal os can be reattempted right after the injections. For the overwhelming majority of patients, hysteroscopy will then be painless. If the patient still reports pain after the injection of a total of 10 mL of the anesthetic agent into both sacrouterine ligaments, 5 mL more is directly applied at four to six paracervical points (Fig. 42).

The dosage required depends primarily on the general condition of the patient. Detailed information on the procedure and possible complications beforehand will alleviate anxiety and reduce the need for

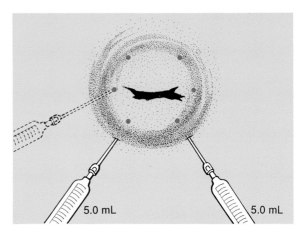

Fig. **42**   Technique of paracervical block

analgesia. We have also found it helpful to talk with the patient during the procedure. Ideally, the patient can follow the procedure on a video monitor, and further explanations can be given as it progresses.

Learning Hysteroscopy

Like any other invasive procedure, hysteroscopy must be learned. However, the most difficult step of the procedure—passing the internal os of the uterus—is performed by any gynecologist during conventional dilation and curettage.

Possible Difficulties

a) **The uterine cavern does not unfold.** If the tip of the scope is in the uterine cavity, it can usually be surveyed without difficulty. If this is not the case, the hysteroflator, gas flow, and intrauterine pressure should be checked. If the flow is normal, there may be a leak in the working sheath or in the gas-conducting tubing. This can be evaluated by removing the tip of the hysteroscope from the uterus and immersing it in liquid (sterile saline or, during outpatient hysteroscopy, in chlorhexidine gluconate solution) (Fig. **43**). Normally, bubbles should flow rapidly from the tip of the scope. If not, and if the flow is high, a leak should be looked for in the gas-conducting tubing and in the connection between the hysteroscope and the sheath. If the flow is low, the shaft may be partially occluded by clotted blood (although this seldom occurs with modern sheaths). To remove such particles the sheath is rinsed with 5 mL of saline.

We have found it useful to check the gas supply at the beginning of the procedure by dipping the tip of the scope into a liquid (Fig. **43**).

b) **Endometrial bleeding is heavy enough to obscure vision** (Fig. **44**). First, wait a few seconds. Often, the intracavitary pressure presses the blood to the uterine wall, and a good view becomes possible. Similarly, bubbles often form and impede or prevent vision. Here too the examiner should wait and move the hysteroscope slowly back and forth to disperse the bubbles. Blood and mucus can form deposits directly on the optical system and partially or completely block vision. In these cases, rubbing the tip of the hysteroscope in the uterine fundus often removes such deposits (as at laparoscopy). If not, the hysteroscope has to be removed and its tip cleaned with a swab.

Learning hysteroscopy takes patience. Early in our experience, we needed 5 minutes or longer for one study; now we average 1 to 2 minutes. Patience is needed during individual examinations when the examiner is waiting for bubbles or blood to clear and during series of examinations, for example when

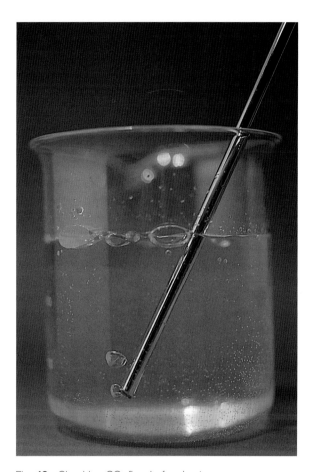

Fig. **43**   Checking CO_2 flow before hysteroscopy

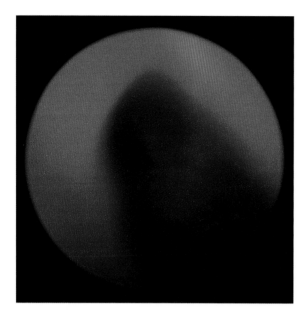

Fig. **44** Visibility impaired by blood

10 consecutive procedures fail to yield satisfactory results. In the latter case, we recommend watching an experienced hysteroscopist at work and then, with his or her help, beginning anew. From working with colleagues visiting our clinic to learn hysteroscopy, we have found that small details usually disturb the examination. However, small problems can become so irritating that some colleagues have nearly rejected the method altogether.

Generally, it takes about 50 hysteroscopies to become dexterous enough with the technique that problems either no longer arise or can be dealt with immediately. For physicians in training, we recommend learning hysteroscopy by performing it in patients under general anesthesia for subsequent curettage. For practicing gynecologists, we recommend spending some time with an experienced hysteroscopist to become familiar with the technique before investing in a hysteroscopy unit. Then, after collecting some firsthand experience, it helps to talk over any problems that may have come up with an experienced colleague and perhaps again watch him or her at work.

Investigation of the Endometrium

Studies of the endometrium have long been a major focus of hysteroscopy, and the literature on the diagnosis of endometrial abnormalities is extensive (Schmidt-Matthiesen 1966; Marleschki 1968; Lindemann 1975; Hepp 1977; David et al. 1978; Lübke 1983; Deutschmann and Lücken 1984; Dexeus et al. 1984; Gimpelson 1984; LaSala et al. 1984; Wamsteker 1984; Van Herendael et al. 1987; Mencaglia et al. 1987). Most of these authors have reported high degrees of accuracy.

The goal of hysteroscopic evaluation of the endometrium is primarily to distinguish normal changes from carcinomas and their precursors. But the appearance of the endometrium depends on numerous endogenic and exogenic influences. By taking a careful history, the hysteroscopist can make a picture of the type of endometrium to be expected.

For example, one would expect a carcinoma in an elderly patient with heavy bleeding; hyperplasia, a polyp, or nonfunctional endometrium in an early menopausal patient with atypical uterine bleeding; and normally developed mucosa appropriate for the phase of the cycle in a patient with a lost IUD.

The differential diagnostic assessment of the appearance of the endometrium requires a knowledge of endometrial histopathology (Table 15).

Table **15**

	Endometrial histology according to menopausal status		
	Premenopause	Menopause	Postmenopause
Benign findings	Proliferation	Poor proliferation	
			Resting endometrium
	Secretory transformation		Atrophy
	"Oral contraceptive endometrium"		
	Juvenile hyperplasia		Glandular-cystic (simple or complex) hyperplasia
			Endometrial polyps
Precursors of malignancies			Adenomatous (atypical) hyperplasia Grade 1 Grade 2 Grade 3
Malignancies	(Adenocarcinoma)		Adenocarcinoma

Pathology of the Endometrium

Prerequisites for Hysteroscopic and Histologic Endometrial Diagnostics

For the histopathologist it is often difficult to make a definitive diagnosis on endometrial biopsies if relevant clinical findings have not been communicated completely. This also applies to hysteroscopy. Depending on the patient's age and history, a hysteroscopic or histologic finding can have completely different implications.

A nonfunctional endometrium in a 25-year-old woman has to be judged differently from one in a 53-year-old woman, though the histologic findings may be identical. Progestin therapy can cause endometrial changes similar to those of extrauterine pregnancy. Thus, the hysteroscopist must know whether a patient has been receiving hormone therapy and if so, at what dosages.

A reliable diagnosis of hysteroscopic and histologic endometrial findings requires knowledge of the following patient information:

1. Age
2. Menopausal status
3. Cycle data and day of the cycle
4. Exogenous hormone treatment (medication(s), dosage, duration)

Hysteroscopic diagnosis of endometrial findings requires knowledge of the appearance of normal and abnormal states of the endometrium and of endometrial histopathology. In particular, it is important to be able to distinguish malignant tumors and their precursors from insuspect changes.

The following sections describe the basics of the histopathology of the endometrium. Special attention is paid to functional processes and the transitions between individual normal and abnormal conditions. All endometrial findings relevant to hysteroscopy are discussed from a morphologic point of view. Readers interested in further details are referred to specialized textbooks (Dallenbach-Hellwig et al. 1983, 1984; Hendrikson-Kempson 1980; Kurman 1987).

Normal Types of Endometrium

Before menopause, the proliferating endometrium during the first half of the menstrual cycle and the secretory endometrium during the second half are the normal states of the uterine mucosa. After menopause, inactiv or atrophic endometrium is the norm. In between, there are variants of premenopausal and postmenopausal endometrium caused by the hormonal transition of early menopause.

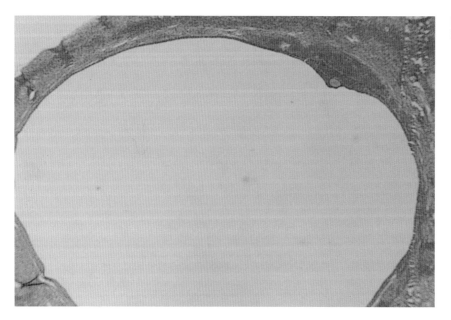

Fig. **45** Graafian follicle just before ovulation

Fig. **46** The wall of a mature follicle with granulosa and theca cells

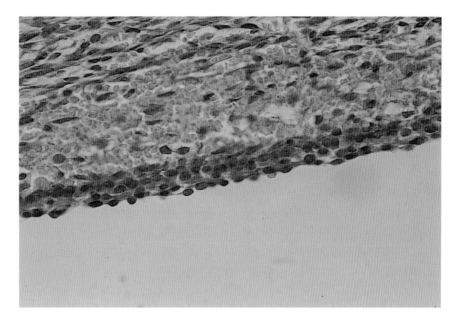

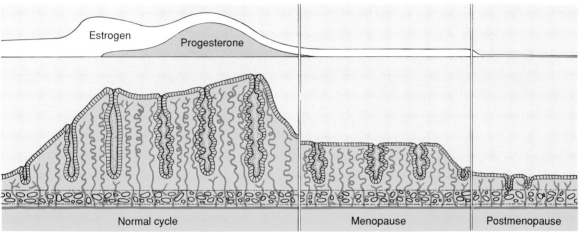

Fig. **47** Schematic representation of the physiological endometrial architecture during various phases of the cycle and phases of life

The Regular Menstrual Cycle

According to ovarian function, the cycle is divided into the follicular (proliferative) phase and the luteal (secretory) phase. During the follicular phase, the granulosa and theca cells (Figs. **45, 46**) produce estradiol, which induces proliferation of the endometrium. During the first half of the cycle, the endometrium grows. Numerous mitoses can be seen in the glands as well as in the stroma. In a regular 28-day cycle, the proliferative phase lasts 14 days; it can vary from 10 to 20 days without any functional disturbance.

The second half of the cycle normally also lasts 14 days with only slight variations of 1 to 2 days. The luteal (secretory) phase is governed by the corpus luteum, which is formed from the follicle after ovulation. The granulosa cells develop into granulosa lutein cells, which dominate the histologic picture; the theca lutein cells, which develop from the theca cell

layer, form only a thin peripheral layer. The corpus luteum produces progesterone and much smaller amounts of estradiol. Progesterone causes the secretory transformation of the endometrium.

Estradiol and progesterone govern the cycle through specific receptors located in the glandular epithelium and the stroma (Haselbach et al. 1988). Stimulation of the endometrium ceases with the cessation of ovarian function at menopause so that finally only an atrophic mucosa remains (Fig. **47).**

The Proliferative Phase

Since the proliferative phase can vary in duration under normal conditions, histology can give only an estimate of the day of the cycle. An early, a mid, and a late proliferative phase are distinguished.

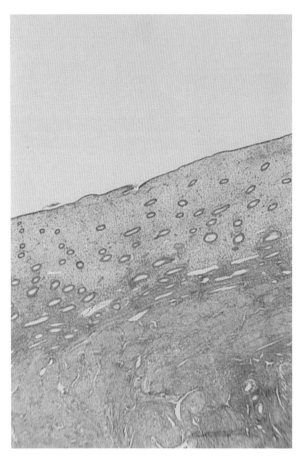

Fig. **48**   Early proliferative phase. HE, x 30

Early Proliferative Phase

In the early proliferative phase, the endometrium is thin. It contains few glands, and its surface appears smooth. The stroma, glands, and blood vessels all proliferate. The glands are stretched; the stroma is spindly and edematous (Fig. **48**).

Mid Proliferative Phase

In the mid proliferative phase, the glands grow more rapidly than the stroma and thus become tortuous. Mitoses, already present in the early proliferative phase, increase in number. The stroma is still spindle shaped but markedly edematous, which increases the height of the endometrium. The surface is still smooth (Fig. **49**).

Late Proliferative Phase

Shortly before ovulation, the complexity of the glands increases further. The mitotic activity is intense, and the glands are now lined with several cell layers. The cells of the stroma are still spindle shaped but somewhat larger than during the mid proliferative phase. Since the interstitial edema is decreasing, the height of the epithelium remains roughly the same despite further growth. The surface is still smooth (Fig. **50**).

During the entire proliferative phase, immunohistochemistry shows high concentrations of both

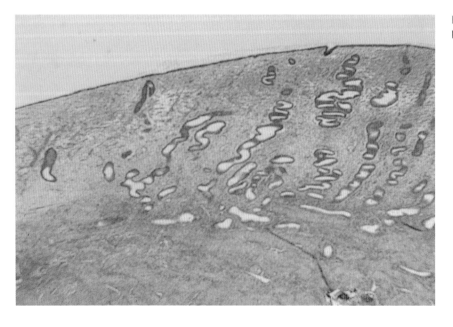

Fig. **49**   Mid proliferative phase. HE, x 30

estrogen and progesterone receptors in the glands and the stroma (Fig. **51**). The surface epithelium does not contain receptors (Fig. **52**).

Secretory Phase

In the absence of endocrine abnormalities, the secretory phase lasts exactly 14 days. Progesterone affects such specific endometrial changes that histology of an endometrial sample can make an accurate diagnosis of the day of the cycle and detect functional abnormalities reliably. Consequently, histologic investigation of dysfunctional bleeding should always be performed during the second half of the cycle.

The day-to-day histology of the secretory endometrium is beyond the scope of this book. However, like the proliferative phase, the secretory phase can be divided into three subphases.

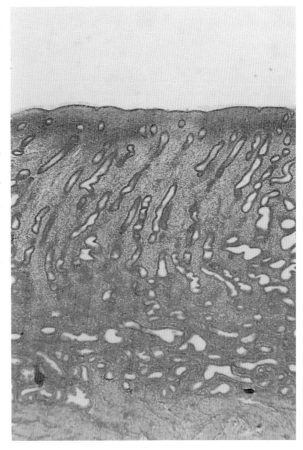

Fig. **50**   Late proliferative phase. HE, x 30

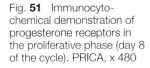

Fig. **51**   Immunocyto-chemical demonstration of progesterone receptors in the proliferative phase (day 8 of the cycle). PRICA, x 480

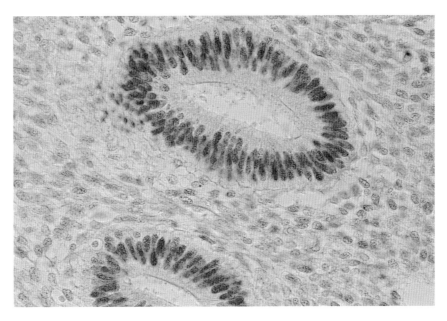

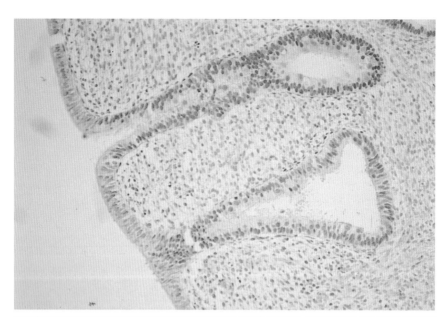

Fig. **52**   Receptor-negative surface epithelium of the glandular excretory duct. A strong positive reaction extends up to the level of the orifice. PRICA, x 220

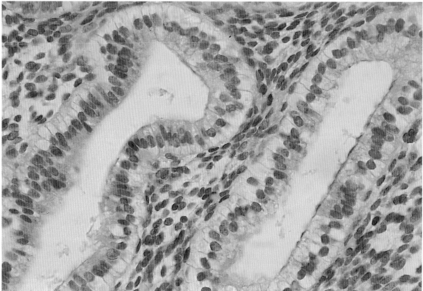

Fig. **53**   Retronuclear vacuoles in the early secretory phase. HE, x 480

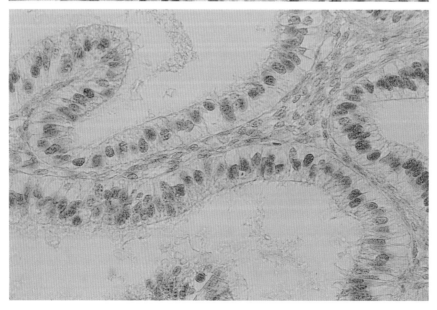

Fig. **54**   Immunohistological study of the endometrial glands in the early secretory phase (day 17). The nuclei are positive for estrogen receptors. ERICA, x 480

Fig. **55** Glandular excretory duct in the proliferative phase. The lumen is relatively small, HE, x 75

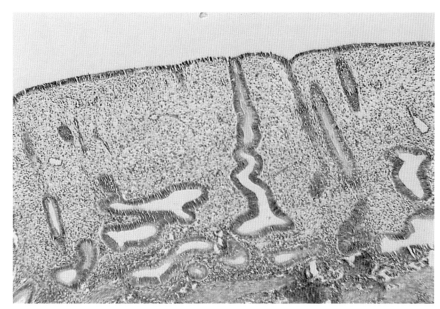

Fig. **56** Glandular excretory duct in the secretory phase. The orifice of the gland is funnel shaped. HE, x 75

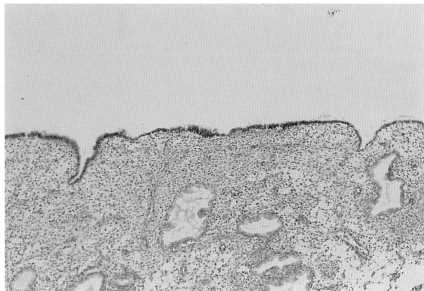

Postovulatory Phase
(1 to 4 days after ovulation)

About 2 days after ovulation, vacuoles, so-called retrovacular translucencies, appear in the bases of the glandular epithelial cells (Figs. **53, 54**). These are seen in almost all columnar cells until the 4th postovulatory day. The glands themselves are tortuous and somewhat wider than during the late proliferative phase. The stroma is unchanged; mitoses are no longer seen in the glands or stroma. The surface is smooth, but the glandular excretory ducts appear wider than during the first half of the cycle (Figs. **55, 56**). The height of the endometrium has increased slightly compared to the late proliferative phase (Fig. **57**).

Mid Secretory Phase
(5 to 9 days after ovulation)

Vacuole formation has now extended to the apical part of the glandular cells, and the nuclei have returned to the base of the cells. Signs of active secretion are seen: the apical cytoplasm border loses its smooth contour, and the glands are increasingly swollen by intraluminal secretion. The glandular ducts become increasingly tortuous.

Seven and eight days after ovulation, there is also interstitial stroma edema, so that the endometrium is at its greatest height during this time. The surface is smooth; the glandular excretory ducts are wide (Fig. **58**).

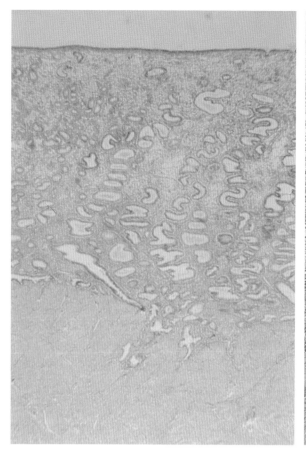

Fig. **57** Early secretory phase. The glands are complex. HE, x 30

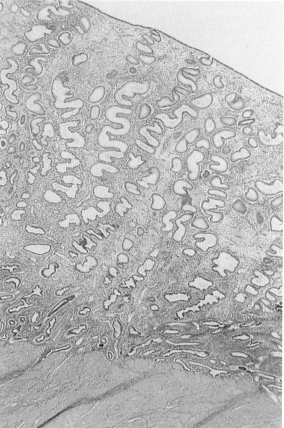

Fig. **58** Mid secretory phase. The height of the endometrium has increased. HE, x 30

Premenstrual Phase
(11 to 14 days after ovulation)

The stromal edema resolves during this phase and the height of the endometrium decreases. Secretion has stopped. The glands themselves remain wide open. The cells of the stroma begin to differentiate into large predecidual cells with round nuclei and small granular cells.

In the late luteal phase, the endometrium consists of the zona functionalis, which is shed during menstruation, and the zona basalis. The zona functionalis consists of the zona compacta, a thick surface layer dominated by stromal cells, and the zona spongiosa, which is dominated by dilated glands (Fig. **59**). The demarcation within the zona functionalis becomes clearer as menstruation nears, and the height of the endometrium decreases markedly.

During menstruation the entire zona functionalis is shed in fragments; only the zona basalis remains and is the source of the endometrium for the next cycle.

During the secretory phase, estrogen and progesterone receptors in the zona functionalis disappear; immunohistochemistry is negative after day 21. Receptors persist in the basal layer, which, upon hormonal stimulation, enters into the next proliferative phase (Riehm et al. 1986) (Fig. **60**).

Atrophy

Atrophic endometrium is characterized by its low height. Glands are sparse, the epithelial cells are pencil-like, the stroma is spindle shaped and mostly compact, and the surface is smooth (Fig. **61**).

Normal Variants of
Atrophic Endometrium

The atrophic endometrium reflects the endocrine milieu. Individual variations are also seen. Complete atrophy does not set in immediately after menopause. First, the height of the endometrium declines morphologically and hysteroscopically. Histologically, glands become scarce even though individual epithelial cells still resemble those of a proliferating endometrium. The stroma is spindle shaped; mitoses are scarce or absent. This picture is often referred to as "functionless" or "resting" endometrium.

Histology also occasionally shows "inferior" proliferation with scattered mitoses and occasional stromal edema. In general, these findings are much less extensive than during a normal proliferative phase.

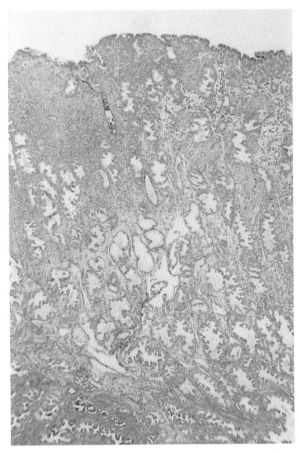

Fig. **59** Late proliferative phase with clear delineation of the zona basalis and the zona functionalis with the zona spongiosa and compacta. HE, x 30

Fig. **60** Endometrium in the late secretory phase with the receptor-negative zona functionalis and the receptor-positive zona basalis on day 27. PRICA, x 30

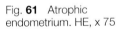

Fig. **61** Atrophic endometrium. HE, x 75

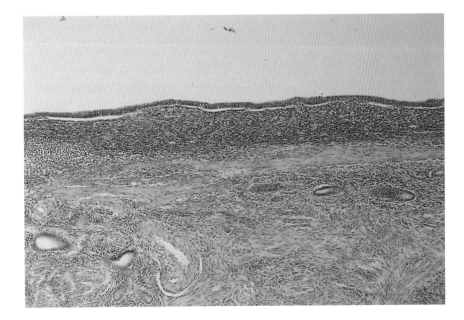

In all these normal variations the surface may not appear totally smooth. It can have irregularities or bumps caused by foci of increased proliferation or localized stromal edema.

Changes Associated with Oral Contraceptives

The endometrial changes in patients taking oral contraceptives depend on the formulation. Although all combination formulations suppress the physiologic development of the endometrium as well as ovulation, single-phasic and multiphasic combinations (which mimic the natural cycle) have different effects on the endometrium.

The height of the endometrium in women taking multiphasic formulations is similar to that in women with normal cycles who are not taking oral contraceptives. However, endometrial height decreases with long-term use. This is compatible with the reports of patients who say that the amount of menstrual bleeding decreases during oral contraceptive intake. These changes set in earlier in patients taking monophasic formulations than in those taking multiphasic oral contraceptives.

Histology then usually shows an irregularly constructed endometrium with rarified glands. The progestin component of the formulation can cause signs of abortive, incomplete secretion in the glands (Fig. **62**). True secretory transformation is seldom seen. The endometrial surface can be either smooth or irregular.

Endometrial Carcinoma and Its Precursors

Carcinogenesis

Endometrial carcinoma occurs primarily in postmenopausal women. Its incidence is increasing in Europe and the United States, and in these areas its prevalence has overtaken that of cervical cancer (Weiss et al. 1976). In Germany, endometrial carcinoma is the most common malignancy of the female genital tract. In contrast, the disease is infrequent in Africa and Asia.

The reasons for this are largely unknown. High-fat diets and longer life expectancies in developed countries probably play a role. In developing countries, many women die before menopause. Unopposed estrogen replacement therapy, which was continued into old age, particularly in the United States, has also been implicated in the increasing incidence of endometrial cancer.

The cumulative 5-year survival rate of patients with endometrial cancer is 70.7%, a relatively good prognosis (Kottmeier 1985). This is because the disease causes atypical uterine bleeding at an early stage in most patients. The prognosis of patients with advanced disease cancer is still poor.

Endometrial carcinoma is a good example of a cancer that can be cured if diagnosed and treated early. However, the endometrium is less accessible than the cervix and prevention of cancer thus more difficult.

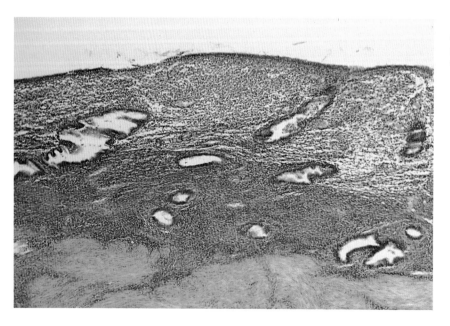

Fig. **62**   Endometrium on day 21 in a patient with a multiyear intake of a triphasic oral contraceptive. HE, x 75

Consequently, there is no generally accepted method for prophylaxis or early recognition of endometrial carcinoma. In the last few years, evidence has been accumulating that there are two groups of endometrial carcinomas with different carcinogeneses and prognoses (Kurman & Norris 1987).

One group of endometrial carcinomas develops via hyperplasia induced by overstimulation of the endometrium by estrogens. These estrogens can be endogenous or exogenous. The first increment of this hyperplasia, glandular or glandular–cystic (simple or complex) hyperplasia, is a completely benign finding. It consists of stimulated glands with no tendency toward autonomous growth. Such hyperplasia is fully reversible after cessation of the stimulus.

But adenomatous (atypical) hyperplasia can develop within glandular–cystic (simple or complex) hyperplasia, particularly under continuing estrogen influence. This represents true glandular neoplasia with cytologic atypia. The risk of progression to carcinoma is associated with the degree of nuclear atypia.

Accordingly, patients found to have glandular–cystic (simple or complex) hyperplasia at fractional curettage require no further treatment whereas those found to have adenomatous (atypical) hyperplasia have been advised to undergo hysterectomy. However, there have been reports that adenomatous (atypical) hyperplasia is completely reversible by progestin therapy (Dallenbach-Hellweg & Schmidt-Matthiesen 1983).

The risk of progression to carcinoma associated with the various hyperplastic lesions of the endometrium is shown in Table **16** (Bonte 1987).

Table **16**   Risk of malignant transformation associated with hyperplastic changes (Bonte 1987)

Glandular (simple) hyperplasia	0.25% –	1.6%
Glandular–cystic (complex) hyperplasia	1.53% –	4.0%
Adenomatous (atypical) hyperplasia, Grade I	15% –	29%
Adenomatous (atypical) hyperplasia, Grade II	10% –	100%
Adenomatous (atypical) hyperplasia, Grade III		100%

Carcinomas arising from hyperplasias are usually well differentiated and become apparent early on by atypical uterine bleeding. The age peak of patients with these carcinomas is 59 years.

In older women, the mechanism of carcinogenesis due to permanent estrogen stimulation of the endometrium is unlikely. These tumors seem to develop de novo. This hypothesis is supported by the observation that atrophic endometrium is frequently seen in the neighborhood of these carcinomas, whereas areas of hyperplasia are often found near carcinomas presumed to have developed through estrogen stimulation (Zerwas & Neis 1990). Endometrial carcinomas in older women are typically poorly differentiated (Table **17**).

Poorly differentiated carcinomas are generally more aggressive and spread more rapidly, locally and distantly. Consequently, they tend to be diagnosed at more advanced stages and have a poor prognosis.

Table **17**   Carcinogenesis of endometrial carcinoma in perimenopausal and postmenopausal patients

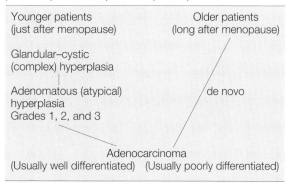

Endometrial Hyperplasias

Glandular–Cystic (Simple or Complex) Hyperplasia

The endometrium is highly built-up and rich in glands, any number of which may be cystically dilated. If there is no cystic dilation, the picture is referred to as glandular or simple hyperplasia. Most glandular ducts are lined with a multilayered epithelium that shows numerous mitoses. The stromal cells are spindle shaped and medium sized (Fig. **63**).

Depending on the intensity and duration of the estrogen stimulus, there are transitions from glandular (simple) to beginning and marked glandular–cystic (complex) hyperplasia. If the stimulus ceases, glandular–cystic hyperplasia is sloughed with bleeding or regresses; the epithelium becomes unilayered or even atrophic. In contrast, endometrial cysts remain. This is called resting or regressive hyperplasia or, when pronounced cysts are present in senility, cystic atrophy (Fig. **64**).

Adenomatous (Atypical) Hyperplasias

Adenomatous (atypical) hyperplasias contain true glandular neoplasia. Three grades are distinguished:

Grade 1

The glands are relatively close together and show a multicolumnar, partially multilayered epithelium. There are numerous mitoses but no atypical nuclei; the stroma is rarefied focally, but generally abundant (Fig. **65**).

Grade 2

The endometrium is rich in glands, and the ducts show an atypical pattern with branching and intraluminal papillae. The stroma is spindle shaped and often sparse.

Grade 3

The endometrium is very rich in glands and the stroma markedly rarefied. The epithelium is multilayered; mi-

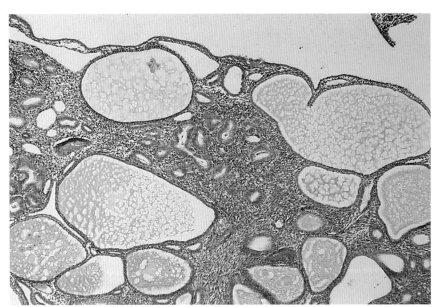

Fig. **63** Glandular–cystic (complex) hyperplasia with cystically dilated, proliferating glands. HE, x 75

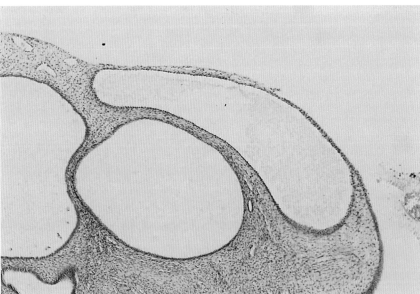

Fig. **64** Cystic atrophy. Only atrophic epithelium is left in cystically dilated glandular ducts. HE, x 75

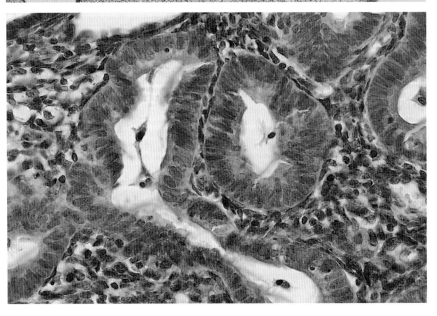

Fig. **65** Adenomatous (atypical) hyperplasia, grade I. This represents true glandular neoplasia with multilayered epithelium and rarification of the stroma. HE, x 480

Fig. **66** Adenomatous (atypical) hyperplasia G3. The cytoplasm is translucent and there is nuclear atypia. HE, x 480

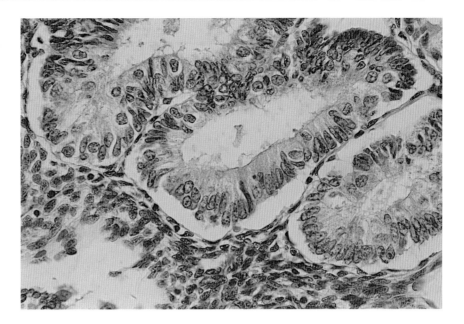

toses are frequent; and the nuclei show atypia at least focally (Fig. **66**).

Grade 3 adenomatous (atypical) hyperplasia used to be referred to as carcinoma in situ of the endometrium. This concept has been abandoned because it was often confused with invasive adenocarcinoma limited to the endometrium. The latter is an invasive endometrial carcinoma that has not yet infiltrated the myometrium. Carcinoma in situ of the endometrium, like that of the cervix, has not breached the basal membrane; these are intraepithelial neoplasias without invasive character.

Invasive Carcinoma of the Endometrium

The degree of histologic differentiation, the depth of invasion into the myometrium, and occasionally the histologic type are important prognostic factors in endometrial carcinoma (Lohe & Baltzer 1981).

The histologic classification for endometrial cancer has been defined by the International Society of Gynecological Pathologists. Three degrees of differentiation are defined, based on histologic and cytologic criteria.

Table **18**   Frequency and prognosis of histologic types of endometrial carcinoma

	Frequency	5-year survival rate
1. Adenocarcinoma		75%
Grade 1 (FIGO): glandular		93%
Grade 2: partly glandular		
partly solid	60%	76%
Grade 3: solid		61%
secretory	1.5%	87%
2. Adenocancroid	21%	87%
(Glandular with benign squamous epithelial metaplasia)		
3. Adenosquamous carcinoma		
Glandular solid (with atypical squamous epithelial metaplasia)	6.9%	47%
Mucoepidermoid (with monocellular mucification and cornification)		
4. Clear cell carcinoma	5.7%	35%
Glandular or papillary		
5. Papillary carcinoma	4.7%	51%
(over 50 % papillary structures)		
Grades 1, 2, 3		

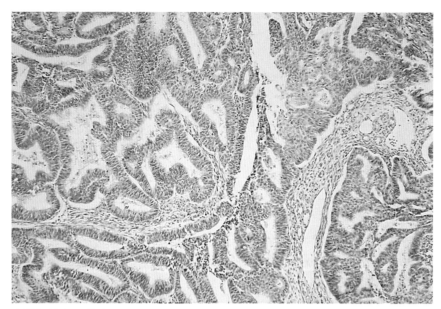

Fig. **67**   Highly differentiated endometrial carcinoma (grade 1) with predominantly tubular growth. HE, x 75

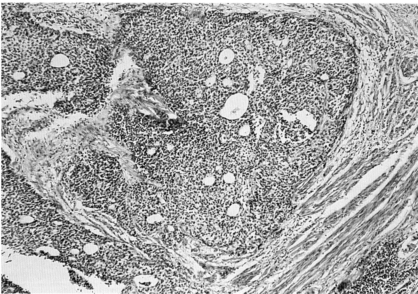

Fig. **68**   Undifferentiated endometrial carcinoma (grade 3). Tumor growth is solid, and there is pseudo-rosette formation. HE, x 75

Grade 1 Adenocarcinoma

These lesions are well differentiated. The glands grow in tubular shapes and are lined with multilayered epithelium. The epithelium shows nuclear anomalies and mitoses; the stroma has vanished, and the glands are packed dos-à-dos (back-to-back) (Fig. **67**).

Grade 2 Adenocarcinoma

Moderately differentiated adenocarcinomas contain well-differentiated compartments as well as solid formations without gland formation.

Grade 3 Adenocarcinoma

Undifferentiated lesions are predominantly solid. Its origin as an adenocarcinoma is often recognizable only by "pseudorosettes," small lumina surrounded by a row of nuclei arranged like a rosette.

Nuclear atypia is almost always more pronounced than in highly differentiated adenocarcinomas of the endometrium. Severe atypias are seen practically only in undifferentiated carcinomas (Fig. **68**).

Special Histologic Types

Adenocancroid and Adenosquamous Carcinoma

These tumors have squamous epithelial elements, which are of metaplastic origin, along with malignant glandular structures. If the squamous epithelial elements are mature and benign, lesions are referred to as adenocancroids or adenoacanthomas (Fig. **69**). If the squamous epithelial component is malignant, the tumor is called an adenosquamous carcinoma. The prognostic significance of squamous epithelial meta-plasias is controversial, but malignant transformation of the squamous epithelial component has been associated with an unfavorable prognosis (Dallenbach-Hellwig & Schmidt-Matthiesen 1983).

Papillary Carcinoma

This lesion (Fig. **70**) is unique in that the prognosis is usually considerably poorer if more than half of a tumor shows papillary differentiation. This applies to all degrees of histologic differentiation (Christopherson et al. 1982).

Clear Cell Carcinoma

This lesion is also associated with a poor prognosis (Fig. **71**). The histologic picture is characterized by large bodies of cytoplasm that appear clear. Most of the nuclei are eccentric (Christopherson et al. 1982).

Fig. **69** Adenoacanthoma with malignant adeno-matous and benign squamous epithelial elements. HE, x 190

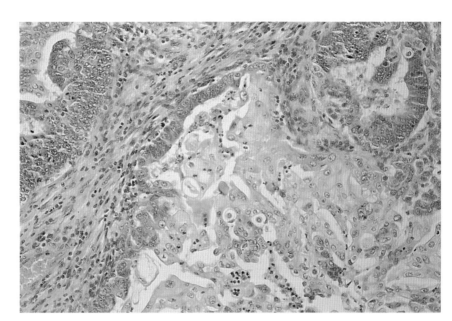

Fig. **70** Papillary endo-metrial carcinoma. HE, x 190

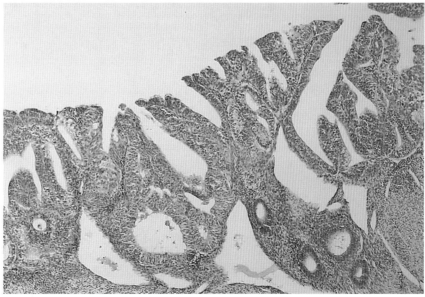

Nonepithelial Tumors

Only a small percentage of endometrial malignancies are nonepithelial. These tumors originate in the endometrial stroma or are mixed, containing mesenchymal, epithelial, and other heterologous components.

Homologous stromal sarcoma, which originates in the endometrial stroma, is the most frequent nonepithelial endometrial tumor. Histology shows mostly uniform spindle-shaped cells. The degree of malignancy depends on the number of mitoses per high-power field. This permits a subclassification that correlates with the prognosis.

Mixed tumors, which contain both mesenchymal and epithelial components, are rare. The tumors are called adenosarcomas if the glandular elements are benign, and carcinosarcomas if both the mesenchymal and the epithelial components are malignant. The classic mixed müllerian tumor also contains heterologous structures such as cartilage, bone, or striated muscle.

Adenocarcinoma of the Endometrium before Menopause

Endometrial adenocarcinoma is extremely rare in premenopausal women under 40. Almost all such tumors are highly differentiated tumors and have good prognoses (Kurman & Norris 1987). The histologic diagnosis of endometrial adenocarcinoma in premenopausal patients—i. e., its delineation from hyperplasia—is difficult.

Accordingly, progestin therapy often leads to complete resolution of the findings. Nonetheless, young patients with invasive endometrial carcinoma should be treated surgically because individual observations have shown that disease can progress rapidly.

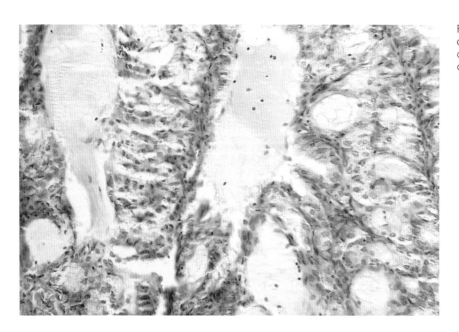

Fig. **71** Clear cell carcinoma with characteristically clear cytoplasm. HE, x 190

Hysteroscopic Differential Diagnosis of the Endometrium

Hysteroscopic diagnoses of endometrial changes are based on the appearance of the surface and the thickness of the mucosa. Certain findings are appropriate for a patient's age and menstrual status; other findings are suspect. Endometrial polyps and carcinomas can practically always be differentiated from normal findings and suspect lesions (Table **19**).

Hysteroscopic Findings before Menopause

Proliferating Endometrium

Proliferating endometrium is characterized by its smooth surface and is yellow-white in color. The surface shows no or only minimal roughness, and the uterine cavity is evenly lined (Figs. **72, 73**). At the beginning of the proliferative phase, both tubal angles are well visible (Fig. **74**). This becomes difficult at midcycle, when the endometrium is thicker.

Secretory Endometrium

The hysteroscopic picture at the beginning of the secretory phase is identical to that in the late proliferative phase; the two cannot be distinguished hysteroscopically.

In the early and mid secretory phase, the endometrium is thick. Its color is yellow, sometimes nearly white. The surface is usually smooth, but particularly in the late secretory phase, polypous endometrial changes and bridges between the anterior and posterior uterine walls can be seen. Hysteroscopy shows wide open glands relatively early in the secretory phase; this permits a rough differentiation between the proliferative and secretory phases (Figs. **75, 76**).

Hysteroscopic Findings in Patients Taking Oral Contraceptives

The appearance of the endometrium depends on the type of oral contraceptive and on how long it has been taken. Here too, the surface is usually smooth, but it can show areas of slight irregularity. The color is white to yellow (Figs. **62, 77, 78**).

Hysteroscopic diagnoses during different phases of life		
Premenopause	**Perimenopause**	**Postmenopause**
Normal Endometrium appropriate for cycle phase	Flat endometrium → Flat and smooth	→ Flat and irregular Atrophy
Carcinoma Suspicious	Thick endometrium → Thick and flat	→ Thick and irregular
	Endometrial polyps Endometrial carcinoma	

Table **19**

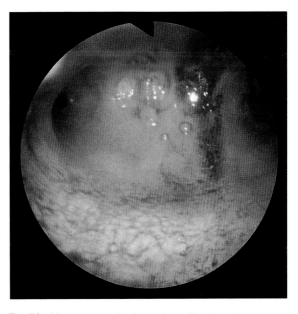

Fig. **72** Hysteroscopy in the early proliferative phase

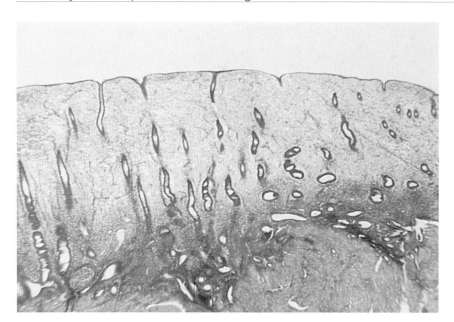

Fig. **73** Early proliferative phase. The surface is smooth, and the glandular ducts are narrow

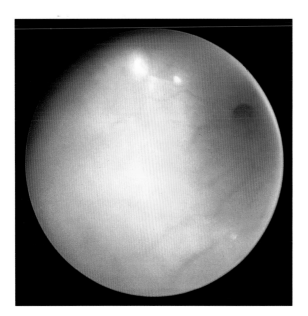

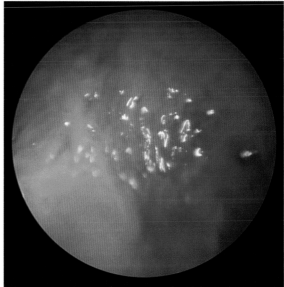

Fig. **74** Hysteroscopic view of the left tubal angle in the early proliferative phase

Fig. **75** Surface of the endometrium in the secretory phase. The glandular ducts are relatively wide

Fig. **76** Histology of the endometrium after secretory transformation. The surface is smooth, and the excretory ducts are relatively wide

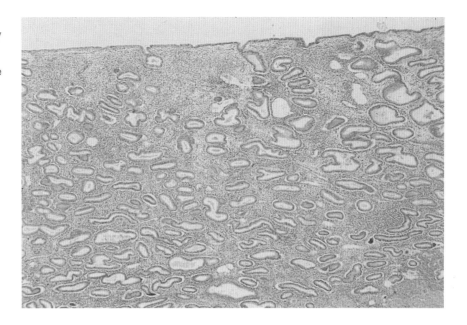

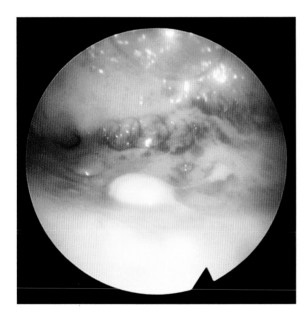

Fig. **77** Hysteroscopic findings in a patient taking an oral contraceptive. There are a few bumps

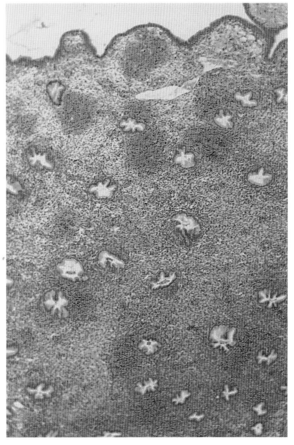

Fig. **78** Histology of the endometrium in a patient taking an oral contraceptive. The surface is slightly irregular

Postmenopause

Atrophy

The normal atrophic endometrium during postmenopause is flat. Its surface is usually smooth, occasionally somewhat irregular. The color ranges from white to yellow, and is sometimes brownish (Figs. **61, 79, 80**). In a uterine cavity lined with atrophic endometrium, the ostia of the tubes are easily visible. They appear perfectly round and rigid. Sometimes the endometrium covers the tubal opening like a veil (Fig. **81**).

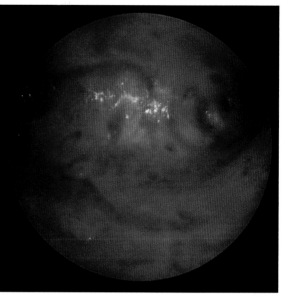

Fig. **79** Hysteroscopic view of atrophic endometrium

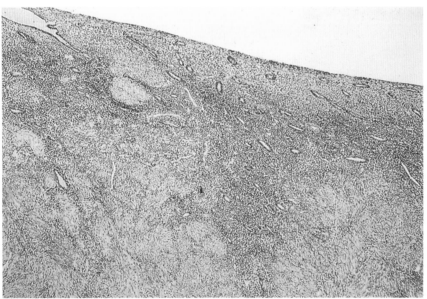

Fig. **80** Histology of complete endometrial atrophy. The surface is smooth, and the glands are rarefied.

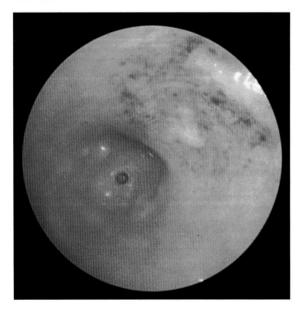

Fig. **81** Rigid tubal angle with atrophic endometrium

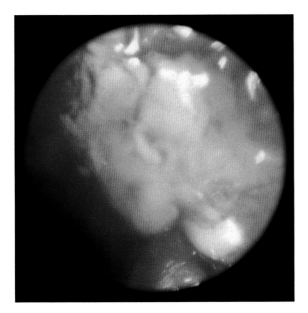

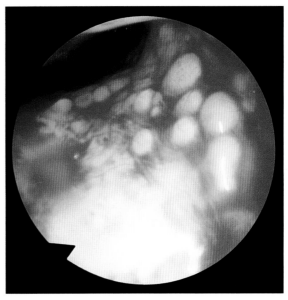

Fig. **82** Flat, irregularly structured endometrium

Fig. **83** Focal color changes of the endometrial surface

Irregularly Structured Endometrium

We distinguish flat and thick irregularly structured endometrium. Both have an uneven surface and depressions and polypous endometrial protrusions. The color of the surface is usually yellow to brown, but can also be white. Sometimes foci of different colors are seen (Figs. **82, 83**).

Flat, Irregularly Structured Endometrium

This is composed of small folds of endometrium formed by atrophic as well as nonfunctional and weakly proliferating endometrial areas lying close together. The density of the endometrial stroma also varies in these areas. This results in the hysteroscopic picture of an irregular surface (Figs. **84, 85, 86**).

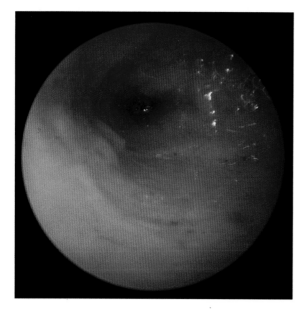

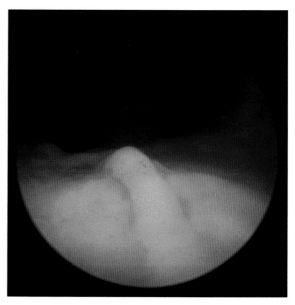

Fig. **84**   Flat endometrium with an irregular surface

Fig. **85**   Fold of a flat, irregularly structured endometrium

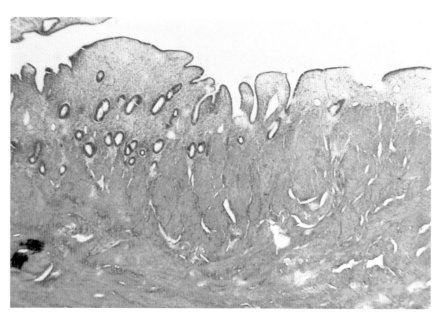

Fig. **86**   Histology of an endometrium with an irregular surface. There are no signs of malignancy or hyperplasia

Thick, Irregularly Structured Endometrium

If the endometrium is thick and its surface uneven, hyperplasia cannot be ruled out by hysteroscopy. Such findings can be due to hormone-replacement therapy with focal proliferation of various degrees or to stromal edema. In these cases deep focal hyperplasias cannot be ruled out. This applies both to lesions covering the entire endometrium and to those limited to a focus (Figs. **87, 88**).

Endometrial Polyps

Endometrial polyps are projections of the mucous membrane; most are broad based, but some are pedunculated. The surface is smooth. Absence of vessels or a delicate vascular plexus suggest a benign polyp. Pellucid cystic structures are sometimes seen (Figs. **89—92**).

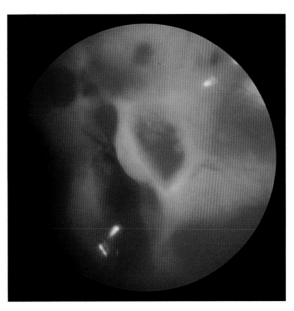

Fig. **87** Thick endometrium with an irregular surface

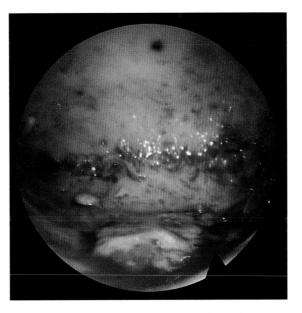

Fig. **88** Panoramic hysteroscopy shows flat endometrium on the anterior wall and foci of thick endometrium on the posterior wall

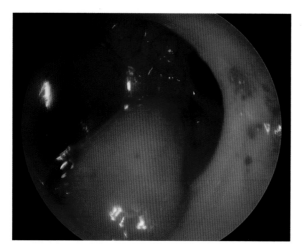

Fig. **89**   Plump endometrial polyp

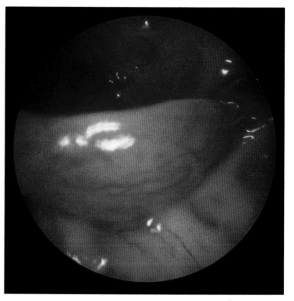

Fig. **90**   Thin endometrial polyp

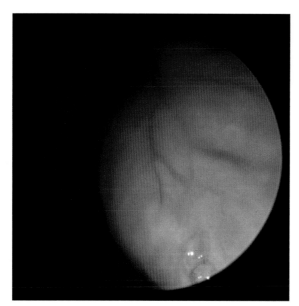

Fig. **91**   Surface of an endometrial polyp with a delicate vascular plexus

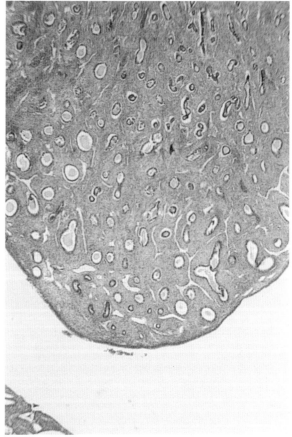

Fig. **92**   Histology of an endometrial polyp. HE, x 30

Fig. **93** Submucosal leiomyoma with a thin endometrial cover

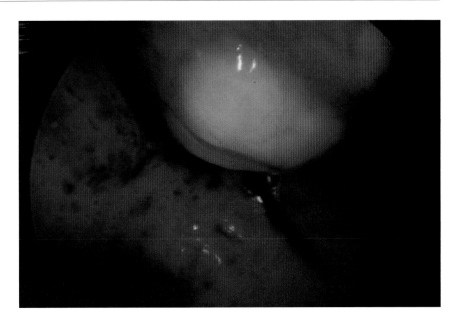

Submucosal Leiomyomas

Endometrial polyps sometimes have to be distinguished from submucosal leiomyomas. Submucosal leiomyomas are usually covered only by a thin layer of endometrium (Figs. **93, 94**). They are usually white to yellow; the base is usually broader than that of an endometrial polyp. Probing the consistency of a lesion with the hysteroscope usually clarifies the situation: submucosal leiomyomas are immobile and much firmer than endometrial polyps.

Hyperplastic Endometrium

Thickened endometrium in a postmenopausal patient always suggests hyperplasia. The surface can be smooth or uneven. Cysts or densely clustered dilated glandular ducts are sometimes seen shining through. The endometrium is much thicker than atrophic or irregularly growing endometrium. Pressure with the hysteroscope leaves an indentation that roughly correlates with the thickness of the endometrium (Fig. **95**). Similarly, pulling the hysteroscope across the uterine wall leaves behind furrows in the endometrium (Fig. **96**).

Hysteroscopy cannot distinguish among the various types of hyperplasia. The hysteroscopist should always proceed under the assumption that every hyperplasia can harbor deep foci of adenomatous (atypical) hyperplasia or an early invasive carcinoma that escape hysteroscopic diagnosis (Figs. **97—100**).

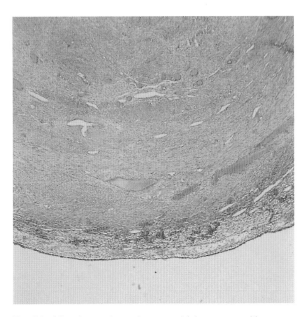

Fig. **94** Histology of a submucosal leiomyoma with pressure-induced atrophy of the endometrium. HE, x 30

This must be taken into account when reporting hysteroscopic findings. Endoscopic inspection cannot provide a definitive diagnosis of a histologic lesion; but the distinction between atrophic and hyperplastic endometrium can be made by a hysteroscopist with little experience.

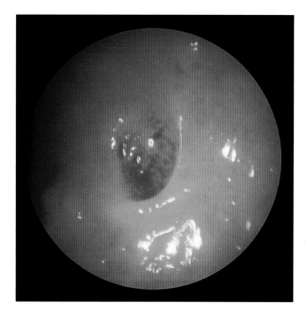

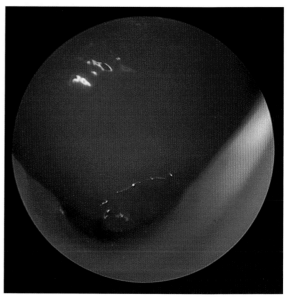

Fig. **95** Indentation of the endometrium made with the hysteroscope. The depth of the indentation corresponds roughly to the thickness of the endometrium

Fig. **96** Furrow in the endometrium

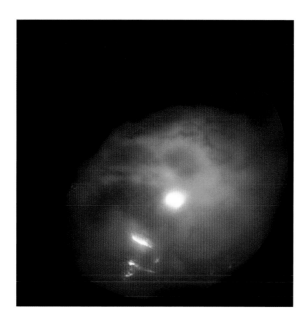

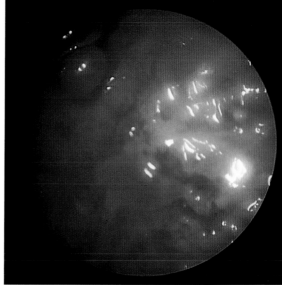

Fig. **97** Glandular–cystic (complex) hyperplasia with cysts shining through

Fig. **98** Glandular–cystic (complex) hyperplasia in an irregularly structured endometrium

Endometrial Carcinoma

Like hyperplasias, adenocarcinomas of the endometrium have a variety of appearances at hysteroscopy. Nonetheless, these appearances are so typical that they are hard to miss. However, hysteroscopy sometimes cannot distinguish between hyperplasia and invasive carcinoma. In these cases, hysteroscopy has done its job when abnormal endometrium has been detected.

Most endometrial carcinomas are polypous tumors with areas of discoloration and necrosis (Figs. **101, 102**). Erratic, large-caliber vessels are often seen on the surface of the tumor, which bleeds easily. If the entire uterine cavity has been occupied by tumor, hysteroscopy is similar to looking into a cave with stalactites and stalagmites (Figs. **103, 104**). The surface of the carcinoma is usually raw and polypous. Some carcinomas have white to yellow surfaces. All endometrial carcinomas are friable and bleed easily when touched.

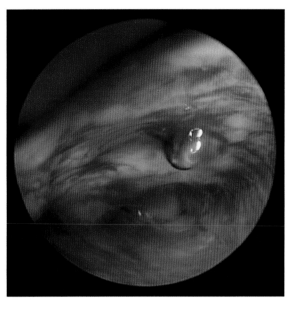

Fig. **99** Irregular, thick endometrium. Hysteroscopy could not rule out carcinoma; histology showed glandular–cystic (complex) hyperplasia

Fig. **100**   Glandular–cystic (complex) hyperplasia in the uterine fundus. HE, x 30

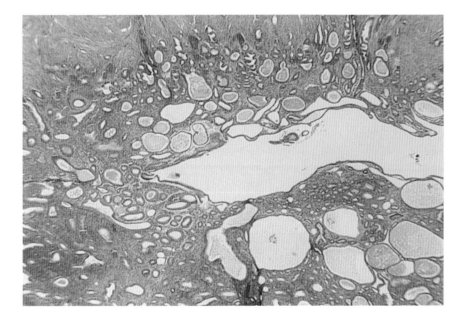

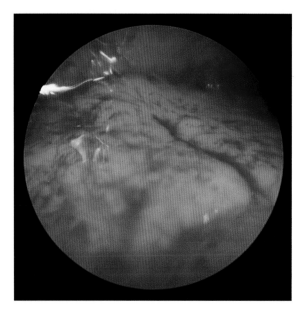

Fig. **101**   Polypous tumor in the uterine cavity with contact bleeding. Histology showed carcinoma limited to the endometrium

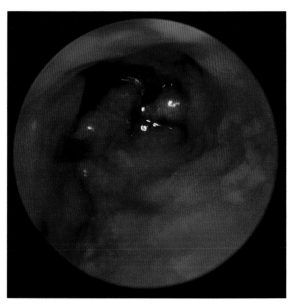

Fig. **102**   Polypous endometrial carcinoma with necroses and blood deposits

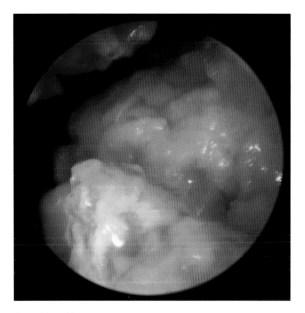

Fig. **103**   Hysteroscopic view reminiscent of a stalactite–stalagmite cave. Histology showed a grade 3 endometrial carcinoma

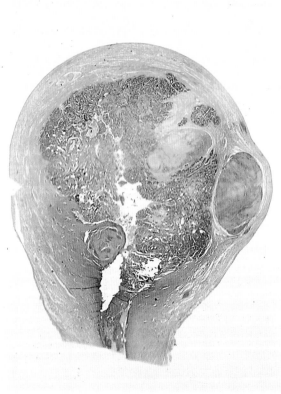

Fig. **104**   Histologic giant section of a uterus (processing technique according to Lohe and Balzer) with an adenocarcinoma of the endometrium

Morphologic Verification of Hysteroscopic Findings in an Outpatient Setting

Hysteroscopic findings can be verified by histology of a biopsy specimen. In turn, a biopsy specimen can be obtained directly under hysteroscopic vision or by streak curettage. Streak curettage can be directed toward a lesion localized at hysteroscopy, or, if the endoscopic findings are homogeneous, a specimen can be obtained from both walls of the cavity.

Biopsy under visual control has the advantage that the suspicious focus is sampled directly. A disadvantage is that the specimen obtained is often so small that an exact histologic diagnosis is difficult. It also requires a hysteroscope with a working channel; the diameter of these instruments is larger and they are not tolerated as well by the patient without anesthesia. These disadvantages led us to quickly abandon biopsy under hysteroscopic guidance, the method we had at first favored. We now perform what we call directed streak curettage.

If hysteroscopy shows findings such as atrophy, representative streaks of tissue are taken from the anterior and posterior walls of the uterus. If a localized lesion is found, a streak is taken from this region. Whereas a small tissue sample suffices if the endometrium is atrophic or flat and irregular, a generous sample is necessary if the endometrium is thick or if carcinoma is suspected (Fig. **105**).

Fig. **105** Endometrium fragment obtained at streak curettage. HE, x 2.5

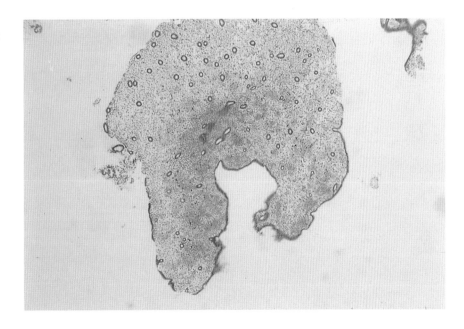

The streak curette we use (Fig. **106**) has a diameter of 4 mm and is thus smaller than the standard 5-mm hysteroscope. Accordingly, we have never had problems passing the cervical canal. Obtaining material is simple and painless if the endometrium is thick. Streak curettage of atrophic endometrium some-times requires pressure to obtain a tissue sample, and some of the patients report brief discomfort. Overall, streak curettage is a quick and simple procedure that is well tolerated. Histologic processing is straightforward and can be performed by any pathology laboratory.

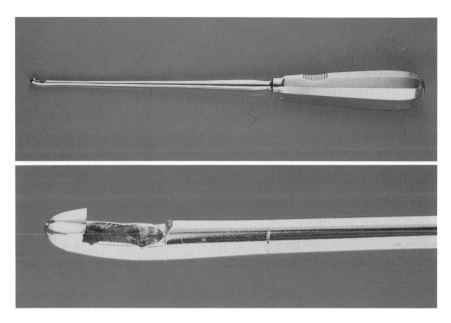

Fig. **106**   Streak curette. The shaft of the instrument is 4 mm in diameter

Cytology of the Endometrium

Cytology of material obtained from the uterine cervix permits early detection of cervical carcinoma and its precursors. The smear is simple to obtain, and the differential diagnosis of the various cervical lesions has been described thoroughly. However, cervical cytology is ineffective for detecting lesions of the endometrium. Even in patients with symptomatic endometrial carcinoma, only 60% of cervical smears contain material from the uterine cavity, and in more than half of these, the tissue is so degenerated that only a presumptive diagnosis can be made (Soost 1980, Neis et al. 1983).

The validity of endometrial cytology has been increased by obtaining material directly from the uterine cavity (Soost 1980, Mencaglia 1987). But the amount of material obtained often also does not suffice for a cytologic diagnosis, and the collection itself can be uncomfortable for the patient (Feichter & Tauber 1981).

Over the years, numerous instruments have been developed for intrauterine cell collection (Gravlee 1969, Jimenez-Ayala et al. 1975, Barbaro et al. 1982, Clocuh et al. 1982, Feichter et al. 1982, Bitsch et al. 1984, Caniels et al. 1985). None of these devices, however, has met all the criteria required for screening purposes: simple handling, painlessness, low cost, accuracy, and low risk. Thus, the series of instruments continues.

A further difficulty with endometrial cytology is that, in contrast to cervical cytology, there are no generally accepted criteria for the various benign and malignant lesions of the endometrium. Although the cytologic findings associated with hyperplasias and carcinomas have been described (Jordan et al. 1956, Boschmann 1958, Berg et al. 1958, Reagan et al. 1973, Ng et al. 1973, Ng 1974, Bibbo 1979), the possibility of recognizing the precursors of endometrial carcinoma has been disputed by other authors (Bachet et al. 1983, Schneider 1985). Thus, endometrial cytology as a whole has been brought into question.

But endometrial cytology has not lost its appeal as a diagnostic technique. Three principle issues have to be addressed:

1. The technique for obtaining a sample
2. The accurancy of detecting hyperplastic and malignant endometrial lesions
3. The differential diagnosis

Techniques for collecting samples. We have studied numerous instruments and techniques for endometrial cytology. Particular attention was paid to the amount and the condition of the material obtained. The Prävikal cell collector (Fig. **107**) had the highest rate of samples judged as abundant (53.3%) and the lowest rate of inadequate samples (2.7%) (Table **20**).

Table **20** Amount of material obtained by various systems for endometrial cytology

Amount of material	Prävikal (n = 100)	Citosmed (n = 100)	Acurette (n = 100)	Abradul (n = 100)
Abundant	53%	36%	37%	39%
Adequate	25%	31%	25%	26%
Little	18%	23%	21%	14%
Inadequate	3%	10%	17%	21%

These results agree with those of other studies (Feichter & Tauber 1981).

The Prävikal system also produced smears that were the least contaminated with blood and thus the easiest to interpret. This may be because the Prävikal, unlike other instruments, has no sharp edges and therefore does not tear large fragments out of the endometrium. The Prävikal was also the easiest system to use and because of its small diameter, tolerated best by the patients. Cell removal immediately follows hysteroscopy; the cells are stained according to Papanicolaou as modified by Bed. We prefer this stain because it seems the best suited for evaluating nuclei, nuclear structures, mitoses, and cytoplasm.

Differential Cytology

We have compared intrauterine smears with the corresponding histologic findings. With experience, we were able to use cytology to assess both the functional status of the endometrium and its benign or malignant nature with increasing accuracy. The high accurancy of endometrial cytology at first surprised even us (Neis et al. 1985).

To work out criteria for endometrial cytology, we examined smears with objectifiable image analyses. The results of these quantitative and semiquantitative studies partially confirmed and objectified our experience (Neis & Rein 1987) (Table **21**).

The size of the nuclei increases and becomes more variable over the spectrum of endometrial conditions from atrophy, proliferation, secretory transformation, and hyperplasia to carcinoma. Carcinomas have the most pleomorphic nuclei although these are also seen,

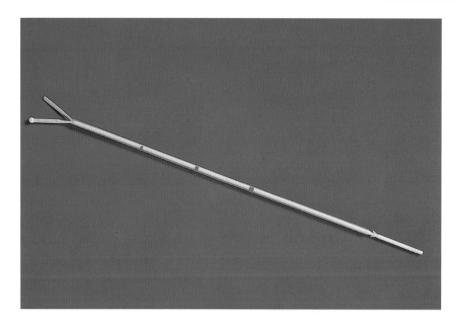

Fig. **107** Prävikal system for obtaining cells from the uterine cavity for endometrial cytology (Nourypharma, Munich)

Table **21**   Criteria of endometrial cytology

	Nuclear size	Nuclei not round	Mitoses	Macro-nucleoli	Visible cell borders	Orderly cell complexes	Dissociated single cells
Atrophy	+	++	-	-	-	+++	-
Proliferative phase	++	-	+	-	-	++	-
Secretory phase	+++	-	-	-	+++	++	-
Hyperplasia	++++	++	++	(+)	+	+	-
Carcinoma	+++++	+++	++	++	-	-	+++

albeit in a much smaller proportion of cells, in hyperplastic conditions. Atrophic endometrium can also show small, pyknic and pleomorphic nuclei.

The number of nucleoli increases with the size of the nuclei. Carcinomas, and some hyperplasias, show macronucleoli. The number of mitoses increases from proliferating endometrium to hyperplasias and carcinomas; atrophic or secretory endometria do not show mitoses. Sharp cell borders in cell complexes are a typical sign of the secretory phase; dissociated, single cells suggest carcinoma. Nearly all other endometrial conditions show more or less orderly cell complexes.

For practicality, we classify our endometrial smears according to a modified Papanicolaou system (Table **22**).

Table **22** Classification of smears obtained from the uterine cavity

	Cytomorphology	Interpretation
E-PAP I	Cell complexes with ordered tissue structure and uniform epithelial cells	Normal endometrium appropriate for cycle phase and age
E-PAP II	Uniform cell complexes with degenerating epithelial cells	Endometrium in desquamation
	Nuclei and cytoplasmic changes suggesting inflammation; round cells and macrophages	Endometritis
E-PAP III	Cell complexes with absent tissue texture and abnormal nuclei; mitoses in postmenopause	Suspicious for hyperplasia
	Degenerated material, material difficult to classify	Unclear findings – hyperplasia or malignancy possible
E-PAP IV	Cell complexes with destroyed tissue texture and small atypical nuclei	Suspicious for atypical hyperplasia
	Isolated severely atypical nuclei	Probable malignancy
E-PAP V	Numerous severely atypical nuclei	Malignancy

Fig. **108** Cytologic specimen with glands and stroma. Papanicolaou, x 75

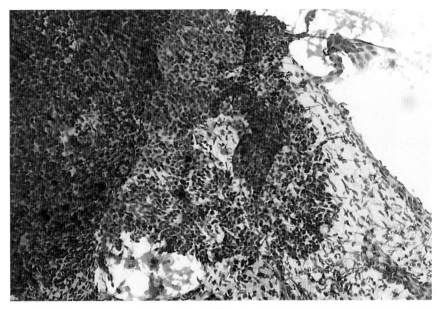

Fig. **109** Glandular epithelium in the proliferative phase with mitoses. Papanicolaou, x 480

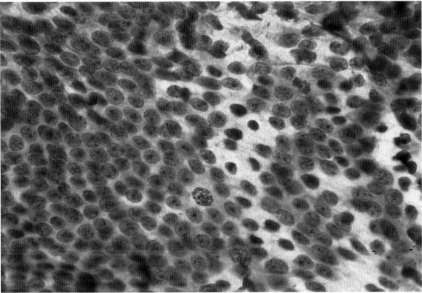

The endometrium consists of glands and stroma. These epithelial and mesenchymal components are usually not difficult to identify in endometrial smears. But the condition of the predominant epithelial component is the issue. Although the stroma also takes part in the cycle, its typical appearance—characterized by spindle-shaped nuclei, basophilic cytoplasm, and an impression of transparency with no visible cell borders—changes little (Fig. **108**).

Proliferating Endometrium

Proliferating endometrium is dominated by orderly cell complexes with small nuclei. The nuclei are relatively close together, but a strip of cytoplasm can usually be seen between cells. The cell borders are blurred. The nuclei appear partly solid, partly loosened, and most contain one nucleolus. Most nuclei are round, but roughly 10% of cells are not completely round. Pleomorphic nucleic patterns are not seen in the proliferative phase, but mitoses are typical for the first half of the cycle and can always be found if looked for (Fig. **109**). Proliferating endometrium can be distinguished from atrophic endometrium by its large nuclei, mitoses, and the somewhat larger amount of cytoplasm.

Secretory Endometrium

Cytology of endometrium in the secretory phase also shows ordered cell complexes. The nuclei are round and loosened and most contain two nucleoli. There are large differences in the size of the nuclei, but the nuclear pattern is otherwise unremarkable. Mitoses are

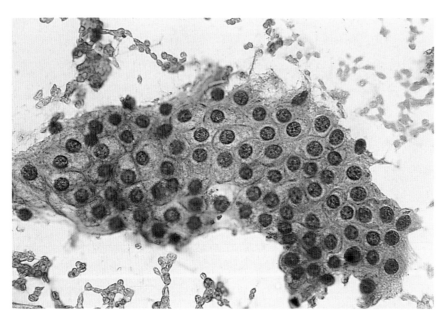

Fig. **110**   Secretory endometrium with sharp cytoplasma borders. Papanicolaou, x 480

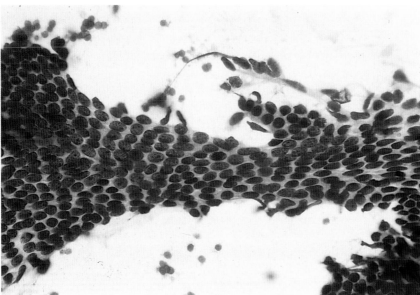

Fig. **111**   Atrophic endometrium. Some of the nuclei are spindle shaped. Papanicolaou, x 480

no longer seen. The cytoplasm is clearly increased compared to other endometrial states and can contain vacuoles. The cell boundaries are clear. The large round nuclei and the abundance of cytoplasm are the most important characteristics of secretory endometrium.

Compared with the proliferative phase, secretory endometrium can be distinguished by the increased amount of cytoplasm, the sharp cell borders, and the absence of mitoses. The nuclei are larger, and nearly all show a loosened internal structure (Fig. **110**).

Atrophic Endometrium

The cells of atrophic endometrium are arranged exclusively in orderly complexes. The nuclei are small; they are partly loosened, partly solid. There are peg-formed

nuclei and pyknic nuclei, some with bizarre forms. Nuclei with a loosened internal structure usually show a small nucleolus. The nuclei are, in general, dense; the cytoplasm is rarefied. Mitoses and macronuclei are absent (Fig. **111**).

Fig. **112**   Endometritis with marked round cell infiltration. Papanicolaou, x 480

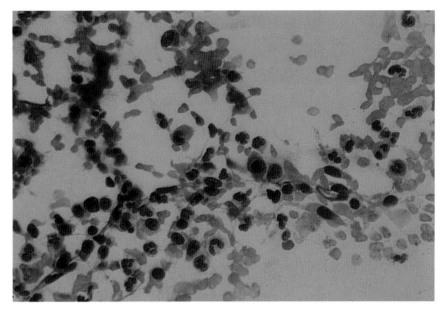

Fig. **113**   Giant cells in a patient with an IUD. Papanicolaou, x 480

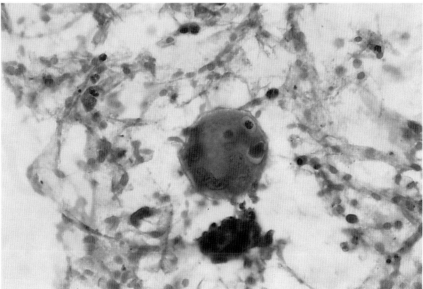

Infection

The appearance of florid endometritis is dominated by round cell infiltration, which permeates the stroma to varying degrees. There are mainly leukocytes with polymorph nuclei plasma cells. The epithelial cells have swollen nuclei, and some have cytoplasmic vacuoles. The background of the specimen usually contains debris (Fig. **112**).

Sometimes there are multinucleated giant cells, which are notable for their large cytoplasm content and their usually eccentric nuclei. These giant cells often are the only sign of an infection in women with IUDs. In these cases, the background of the slide is usually clear; the round cell infiltration of florid endometritis is absent (Fig. **113**).

Degenerative Changes

Endometrium being shed is characterized by swollen cell nuclei and disordered tissue textures. Malignancy can be ruled out if the nuclei are swollen and if polarity is generally preserved (Fig. **114**). However, degenerative changes can be so extensive that hyperplasia or carcinoma cannot be ruled out by cytology alone (Fig. **115**).

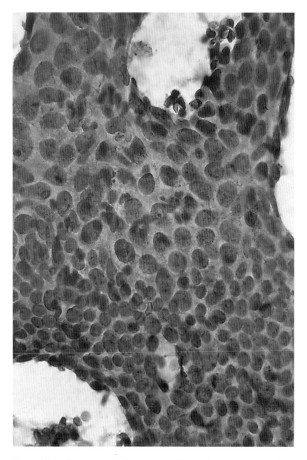

Fig. **114** Degenerated endometrium in desquamation. This smear can barely still be interpreted. Papanicolaou, x 480

Hyperplastic Endometrium

The cytology of endometrial hyperplasia spans the range from glandular–cystic (simple or complex) to adenomatous (atypical) hyperplasia. A cytologic suspicion of hyperplasia should always be followed up with curettage for a definitive diagnosis.

The cells of hyperplastic endometrium are usually in complexes (Fig. **116**); in 30% of samples, the tissue texture has been disturbed. There are large, predominantly round, but also non-round nuclei with a loosened internal nuclear structure. Most nuclei show two nucleoli, some contain macronucleoli. Mitoses are more common than in the proliferative phase; hints of the cell borders remain. Atypical nuclei, if present, are suspicious for adenomatous (atypical) hyperplasia (Fig. **117**).

Hyperplastic endometrium should be distinguished from proliferating endometrium. In contrast to normal proliferation, hyperplasia is characterized by larger nuclei, which are also more often not round. The tissue texture seems less ordered, and nucleoli and mitoses are more common; macronucleoli or atypical nuclei can be signposts. A suspicion of endometrial hyperplasia will also take into account the patient's age, menopausal status, and hormone therapy.

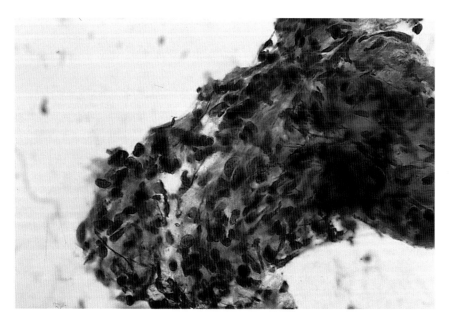

Fig. **115** Degenerated endometrial specimen in a patient with uterine bleeding. No further evaluation is possible. Papanicolaou, x 480

Fig. **116**   Simple glandular-cystic hyperplasia with mitoses. Papanicolaou, x 480

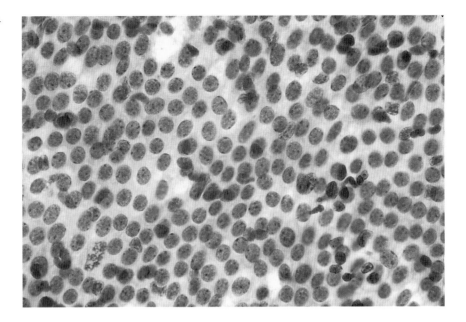

Endometrial Carcinomas and Sarcomas

As in other malignancies, the cytologic appearance of adenocarcinoma of the endometrium is characterized by the abundance of material in the smear. Most cells are dissociated; some are in complexes, which are usually only piles of cells with disturbed tissue texture. The nuclei are considerably enlarged, and according to the degree of differentiation of the tumor, mono-morphic or pleomorphic. Usually, the size of the nuclei varies widely (Fig. **118**).

Nearly all carcinomas with well-maintained internal nuclear structure show nucleoli. Mitoses are always present.

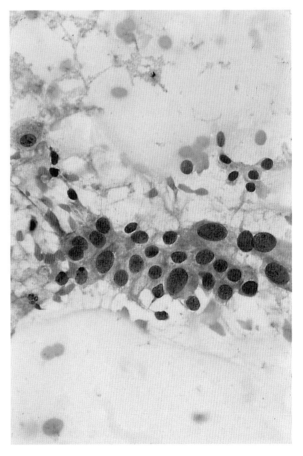

Fig. **117**   Cell complex with atypical nuclei. Histology showed adenomatous (atypical) hyperplasia. Papanicolaou, x 480

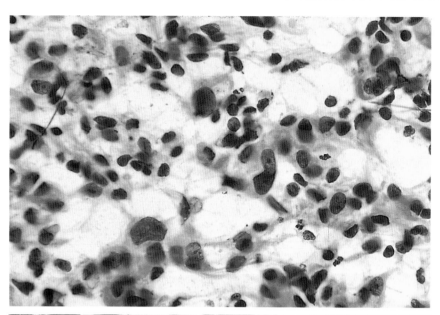

Fig. **118**   Adenocarcinoma of the endometrium with pronounced anisonucleosis. Papanicolaou, x 480

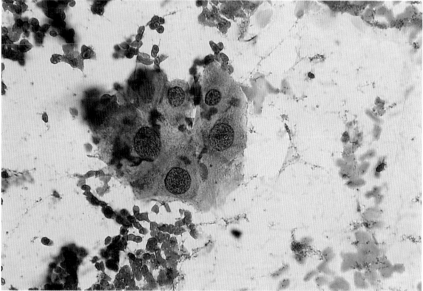

Fig. **119**   Highly differentiated adenocarcinoma of the endometrium with monomorphic but large nuclei. Papanicolaou, x 480

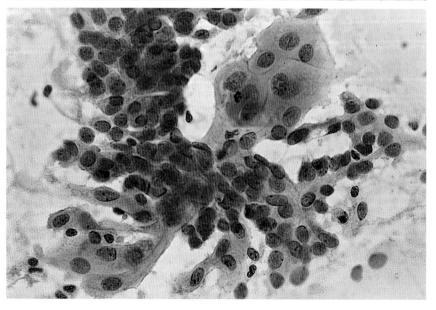

Fig. **120**   Adenoacanthoma of the endometrium with malignant glandular and benign squamous epithelial components. Papanicolaou, x 480

Fig. **121**   Stromal sarcoma with spindle-shaped tumor cells. Papanicolaou, x 480

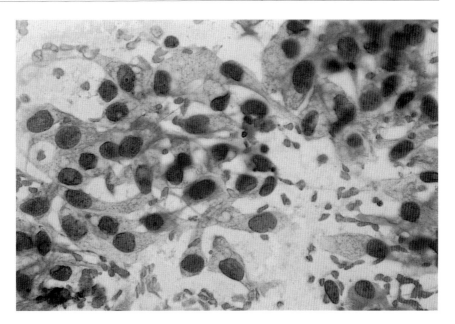

A highly differentiated adenocarcinoma can be difficult to distinguish from (atypical) hyperplasia. The nuclear size and its variability usually suffice for a classification of at least E-PAP IV (Fig. **119**). Occasionally, the histologic type of the tumor is evident, for instance in adenoacanthomas showing malignant glandular and benign squamous epithelial components (Fig. **120**). If only little material is available, or if cytology is made difficult by degenerative changes, the smear is usually classified as E-PAP III. Endometrial sarcomas are rare and show markedly spindle-shaped nuclei, which are usually hyperchromatic and variable in structure and size (Fig. **121**).

Accuracy of Endoscopic and Morphologic Endometrial Diagnostics

Validity of Hysteroscopy

The literature contains numerous reports on the endoscopic diagnosis of endometrial lesions (Schmidt-Matthiesen 1966, Marleschki 1968, Lindemann 1975, Hepp et al. 1977, David et al. 1978, Lübke 1983, Deutschmann & Lüken 1984, Dexeus et al. 1984, Gimpelson 1984, La Sala et al. 1984, Wamsteker & Lücken 1984, Buchholz et al. 1988, Loffer 1989). Most of these authors report high degrees of accuracy, but the results are mostly global so that validity cannot be assessed.

We have compared the histologic results of all our fractional curettages preceded by hysteroscopy with the endoscopic picture. The study consisted of a total of 902 patients (Table 23). Of 43 hyperplasias, only two had been judged normal at hysteroscopy. Both these false diagnoses were made early in our experience. Five patients had hyperplasia hidden in a polyp.

All 87 carcinomas had been classified as abnormal at hysteroscopy. Eighty carcinomas had been classified as such, four were concealed in hyperplasia, and three were contained in polyps.

Minor false diagnoses occurred 23 times. Twenty patients were erronously classified as having hyperplasia and three as having carcinoma.

Thus, the sensitivity of hysteroscopy for detecting hyperplasia or carcinoma was 98.9% with a specificity of 96.7%. The sensitivity for carcinoma only was 100% since all carcinomas were judged abnormal.

Validity of Streak Curettage

The results of complete curettage or hysterectomy were compared with the results of curettage in 437 patients. At first glance, the sensitivity of 69.8% appears somewhat low. One of 87 carcinomas, seven of 35 hyperplasias, and 45 of 48 polyps were not detected. The latter finding is not surprising since a streak curettage cannot remove a polyp.

However, a polyp can hardly be missed at hysteroscopy and is always an indication for complete curettage. Thus, for practical purposes, the validity of streak curettage needs to be evaluated only for hyperplasia and carcinoma. For these conditions combined, the sensitivity of streak curettage was 93.5%. Its specificity was 100%—i.e., there was no histologic overinterpretation (Table 24).

Table **23**   Correlation between hysteroscopy and fractional curettage

Hysteroscopy	Histology					
	Appropriate for phase	Irregular	Polyp	Hyperplasia	Carcinoma	
Appropriate for phase	568	5		②		575
Irregular	46	61				107
Polyp	14	2	53	5	3	77
Hyperplasia	⑬	⑦		36	4	60
Carcinoma		③			80	83
	641	78	53	43	87	902

◯ = False negative   ● = False positive

Table **24**   Correlation between the results of streak curettage and fractional curettage

Streak curettage	Histology					
	Normal	Irregular	Polyp	Hyperplasia	Carcinoma	
Normal	225	5	㊺	⑤	①	281
Irregular	2	35		②		39
Polyp			3			3
Hyperplasia				28	5	33
Carcinoma					81	81
	227	40	48	35	87	437

◯ = False negative

Validity of Endometrial Cytology

In 270 patients, the histologic findings of fractional curettage or hysterectomy were compared with the results of endometrial cytology. All samples for cytology were collected with the Prävikal cell collector. The accuracy of cytology was high: there were only two false positive and two false negative results (Table 25). Two glandular–cystic (simple) hyperplasias were overlooked; one was within and one was next to an endometrial polyp and thus eluded the smear. Both false positive smears came from women who had received radium therapy; cytology showed radiation-induced endometritis.

Again, endometrial polyps were a problem. Of 22 patients with polyps, only three had abnormal cytologic findings. Possible findings are enlarged nuclei in the epithelium covering the polyp (probably due to irritation) or metaplasia. A specific diagnosis was not possible. Half of the patients with endometrial polyps had cytologic findings classified as E-PAP I.

As for streak curettage, the validity of endometrial cytology was evaluated including the polyps and without the polyps. If all pathologic changes (i. e., carcinomas, hyperplasias, and polyps) are included, the sensitivity for detecting carcinomas and hyperplasias was 97.3% and that for carcinomas alone was 100%. The specificity of 84.4% was relatively low because of the E-PAP III results. A finding of E-PAP III means that a carcinoma or a precursor of carcinoma cannot be ruled out. In our series, only half of the patients with a cytology result of E-PAP III had abnormal results at subsequent histology—almost 10% of the entire collective. Here, the limits of endometrial cytology become clear: Applying stricter criteria to avoid false negative diagnoses increases the rate of false positive findings, which in turn decreases specificity.

Validity of the Combination of Hysteroscopy and Streak Curettage

Endometrial cytology has insufficient specificity and thus too many false positive results, particularly in symptomatic patients. Thus, we do not consider it an appropriate technique for the morphologic evaluation of hysteroscopic findings.

Because the sensitivity of directed streak curettage for endometrial cancer is 98.8% and the specificity is 100%, we now use and recommend it in addition to hysteroscopy for all outpatient procedures.

We have compared the results of hysteroscopy plus streak curettage with the final histology results in 438 patients to date (Table 26). There were 13 false diagnoses, but no carcinoma or hyperplasia was missed.

In 474 additional patients, no fractional curettage was performed because endometrial lesions were ruled out by hysteroscopy plus streak curettage. After follow-up of up to 10 years, we have not become aware of a single false negative diagnosis.

Based on these data, the combination of hysteroscopy and directed streak curettage has a sensitivity of 100% and a specificity of 96.2%.

Considering that the sensitivity of "blind" fractional curettage is only 90% to 92% (Schrage 1988), hysteroscopy alone is already superior to the traditional procedure used to investigate atypical uterine bleeding. The combination with directed streak curettage, which usually serves only to confirm the endoscopic finding from a forensic point of view, can clarify unclear cases and detect an occasional false hysteroscopic diagnosis.

In our experience with more than 1000 patients, the sensitivity of hysteroscopy plus streak curettage is 100%. This is uncommon in medical statistics, but not a complete surprise.

Table **25**   Correlation between endometrial cytology and fractional currettage

E-PAP	Endometrium appropriate for age and cycle	Irregular endometrium	Endometrial polyp	Hyperplasia	Endometrial carcinoma	Cervical carcinoma	Total
I	117	12	11	(2)	-	-	142
II	15	2	8	-	-	-	25
III	20	5	3	22	2	2	54
IV	(1)	(1)	-	3	7	4	16
V	-	-	-	-	31	2	33
	153	20	22	27	40	8	270

◯ = False positive ◉ = False Negative

Table **26**   Hysteroscopy and streak curettage

Histology	Normal	Irregular	Polyp	Hyper-plasia	Carci-noma	
Normal	179	13		⑨		201
Irregular	18	44		③	①	66
Polyp			49			49
Hyperplasia			4	30	1	35
Carcinoma			1	1	85	87
	197	57	54	43	87	438

Table **27**   Validity of various techniques for detecting endometrial carcinoma

	Hystero-scopy	Directed streak currettage*	Endometrial cytology*	Fractional curettage**
Sensitivity	100	98.8	97.5	90-92
Specificity	99.5	100	84.4	100

* Neis 1986; ** Schrage 1988

By combining two sensitive techniques such as hysteroscopy and directed streak curettage, one would mathematically expect one false negative diagnosis per several thousand carcinomas. Thus, hysteroscopy plus streak curettage is far superior to fractional curettage, which misses nearly every tenth carcinoma.

Indications for Outpatient Hysteroscopy and for Fractional Curettage

"Any atypical uterine bleeding, especially any bleeding after menopause, is suspicious for carcinoma until proven otherwise." Following this dogma, thousands of curettages are performed every year in Germany. With a million procedures per year, fractional curettage is by far the most frequently performed operation in the United States (Mencaglia 1985). However, the overwhelming majority of these procedures yield normal findings; the real source of the bleeding remains unknown.

Table **28** shows the distribution of findings of diagnostic curettages at our hospital before outpatient hysteroscopy was introduced. Almost 75% of procedures yielded no abnormal findings. In only 23% of the patients did the material collected explain the bleeding and 2.5% of the procedures yielded too little material for a histologic diagnosis.

After it became clear that the combination of hysteroscopy and directed biopsy was very accurate, we increasingly waived fractional curettage if hysteroscopic and morphologic findings were normal. At first we omitted curettage in patients whose medical histories suggested extraendometrial reasons for uterine bleeding (e. g., anticoagulation therapy, cytotoxic chemotherapy, or high-dose gestagen therapy). Then we omitted formal curettage in patients for whom general anesthesia was preferably avoided because of cardiopulmonary risk factors. After finding hysteroscopy

plus biopsy to be accurate and practicable in these patients, we expanded the indications for the procedure to include all patients with atypical uterine bleeding (Neis & Hepp 1985).

If hysteroscopic findings were normal, a streak of endometrium was taken from the anterior and posterior uterine walls to document the hysteroscopic result morphologically. If the two findings agreed, further diagnostics were waived, and the patient was simply followed up. If either hysteroscopy or directed streak curettage yielded abnormal findings, the patient was advised to undergo fractional curettage. Histologic clarification is particularly important in patients with hyperplasia to determine whether the condition is benign, atypical, or malignant. Also, all women with polyps were advised to undergo fractional curettage.

If hysteroscopy suggested carcinoma, a directed streak curettage was performed to confirm the findings. Also, the extent of the carcinoma in the uterus was assessed and curettage of the cervical canal was performed to support the diagnosis. Further clarification with general anesthesia is not necessary before surgery (Table **29**).

Following this procedure, about 60% of the patients are assigned to group I, 30% to group II, and 10% to group III (Table **29**). Thus, about 70% of patients avoid fractional curettage.

Table **28** Results of fractional curettages carried out because of atypical uterine bleeding between 1979 and 1980 at the Department of Obstetrics and Gynecology, University of Homburg (n = 278)

	n	%	Total
Proliferating, secretory, or nonfunctional endometrium	143	51.3	74.5%
Atrophic endometrium	64	23.0	
Endometrial polyp	10	3.6	23%
Glandular-cystic (simple or complex) hyperplasia	20	7.2	
Adenomatous (atypical) hyperplasia	2	0.7	
Adenocarcinoma of the endometrium	32	11.5	
Insufficient material	7	2.5	2.5%

Table **29**   Clinical follow-up after outpatient hysteroscopy

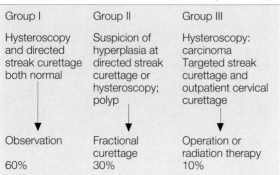

Group I	Group II	Group III
Hysteroscopy and directed streak curettage both normal	Suspicion of hyperplasia at directed streak curettage or hysteroscopy; polyp	Hysteroscopy: carcinoma Targeted streak curettage and outpatient cervical curettage
↓	↓	↓
Observation	Fractional curettage	Operation or radiation therapy
60%	30%	10%

In addition, hysteroscopy can also detect nonendometrial causes of bleeding such as submucous leiomyomas, which are often missed by fractional curettage (Brooke & Serden 1988).

Specific Indications

Intrauterine Staging of Endometrial Carcinoma

In endometrial carcinoma, it is important whether the carcinoma is FIGO Stage I or II. Due to the different routes of lymphatic drainage from the uterine corpus and cervix, different patterns of metastasis must be reckoned with (Lewis & Bundy 1981; DiSaia et al. 1982). An adenocarcinoma that has extended into the cervix may be an indication for a Wertheim-Meigs operation with pelvic lymphadenectomy (Hepp & Neis 1983), whereas a carcinoma limited to the corpus does not require removal of the parametria and the sacrouterine ligaments.

At fractional curettage, the division of the sample into fraction I (cervix) and fraction II (corpus) is supposed to assess the extent of the tumor. Problems arise, however, when tumor is found in both fractions. This may be due to infiltration of the cervix as well as to contamination of the cervical fraction with tissue from the uterine cavity.

We have found that 75% of patients with a positive fraction I at curettage had no infiltration of the cervical mucosa in the hysterectomy specimen (Neis & Schöndorf 1983). In contrast to traditional fractional curettage, hysteroscopy allows an exact assessment of the intrauterine extent of endometrial carcinoma before surgery (Hepp & Roll 1979; Joelsson et al. 1971; Joelsson 1984; Cronje & Deale 1988). Accordingly, we have tried to perform hysteroscopy in all patients referred to our hospital for treatment of carcinoma. A total of 88 patients have been examined; 17 were subsequently treated with radiation therapy so that the hysteroscopic diagnosis could not be checked. In the remaining 71 patients, the preoperative hysteroscopic diagnosis corresponded to the histopathologic findings in the hysterectomy specimen (Table **30**). Carcinoma was limited to the corpus in 66 patients and extended into the cervix in three patients. In nine patients, malignant cells had been found in the cervical fraction of the material obtained at fractional curettage. Hysteroscopy, however, found disease limited to the corpus, so that the stage was revised (Figs. **122—125**).

Overall, the results of hysteroscopic staging agreed with the histologic findings in all patients. Our experience agrees with reports in the literature in which the intrauterine spread of endometrial carcinoma could be predicted accurately in 90% to 100% of patients (Levine & Moberger 1971; Liukko et al. 1979, Baggish 1980).

Table **30** Intrauterine staging of endometrial carcinoma with hysteroscopy (n = 71)

Hysterectomy specimens	71
Agreement between hysteroscopic findings and histopathology	71
Discrepancy between fractional curettage and hysteroscopy (all false positives in curettage)	9

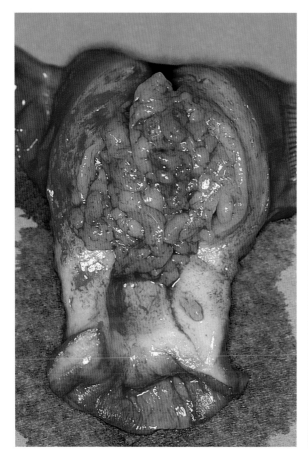

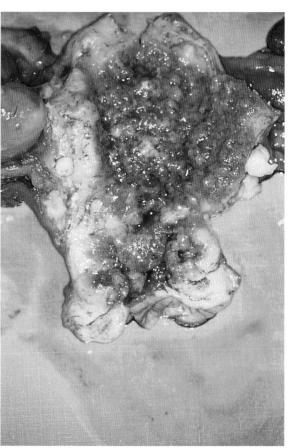

Fig. **122**   Stage I endometrial carcinoma with typical exophytic growth. The cervix is not involved

Fig. **124**   Adenocarcinoma of the endometrium with extension into the cervix (stage II)

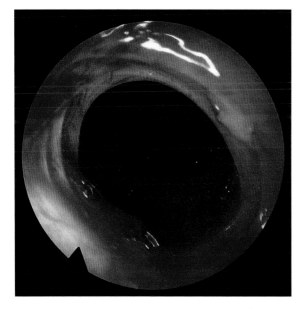

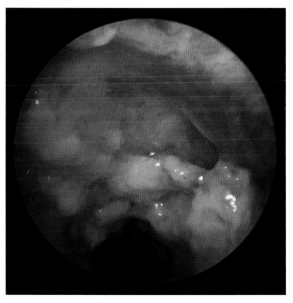

Fig. **123**   Preoperative hysteroscopy of the cervical canal in the same patient. The canal is completely normal

Fig. **125**   Preoperative hysteroscopy of the cervical canal in the same patient. There is clear evidence of malignant infiltration

Follow-Up after Hyperplasia

To evaluate the efficacy of outpatient hysteroscopy for following up patients with endometrial hyperplasia, we reexamined asymptomatic patients in whom simple glandular cystic hyperplasia had been diagnosed within the preceding 3 years. The study included 36 patients who underwent a total of 44 follow-up hysteroscopies. Some of the patients underwent a progestin test at the same time (Noss et al. 1985).

Follow-up hysteroscopy showed complete resolution of the glandular–cystic hyperplasia in 26 patients (Table 31).

Table 31   Follow-up of patient after glandular–cystic hyperplasia (44 hysteroscopies in 36 patients)

Findings	Examinations	Patients	%
Regression (Atrophy)	26	26	70.1
Persisting hyperplasia	10	6	16.2
Progression (endometrial carcinoma)	3	3	8.2
Other (polyps)	5	2	5.4
Total	44	37	100

Six patients had persisting hyperplasia. In two of these, the hyperplasia had resolved at renewed hysteroscopy 3 months later. The four remaining patients underwent two or three further hysteroscopies. Two had glandular–cystic (simple) hyperplasia at subsequent curettage, and two refused the procedure.

Three patients were found to have an asymptomatic endometrial carcinoma. Two of these were adenocarcinomas limited to the endometrium. Streak curettage had shown adenomatous (atypical) hyperplasia in one of these patients and a highly differentiated adenocarcinoma in the other. The third patient refused hysteroscopy; material for endometrial cytology was collected with a Prävikal cell collector and evaluated as E-PAP V. The hysterectomy specimen showed a G1 adenocarcinoma with infiltration into the outer third of the myometrium.

These results suggest that outpatient hysteroscopy with endometrial biopsy is an appropriate follow-up method for patients found to have glandular–cystic (simple or complex) hyperplasia. Regression of hyperplasia can be expected in about 70% of patients. Patients with persisting hyperplasia should be examined at short intervals, possibly after progestin therapy.

Hysteroscopy and endometrial biopsy can detect progressing conditions so that these patients can undergo hysterectomy. If hysteroscopy is not possible, an intrauterine smear should be obtained in all cases.

"Lost" Intrauterine Device

The "lost" intrauterine device (IUD) is a classic indication for hysteroscopy (Hepp 1977, Mohr and Lindemann 1977, Lücken & Lindemann 1977, Gallinat et al. 1978, Wagner 1983, Moulay & Zahi 1983, Tadese & Wamsteker 1985, Burmucic et al. 1987, Assaf et al. 1988). We have had 82 such patients referred to us; in all of these patients, a previous attempt at extraction had been unsuccessful (Table 32). After ultrasound has confirmed that the IUD is in the uterine cavity and ruled out an early pregnancy, hysteroscopy is performed (Fig. 126). When the IUD has been located, the hysteroscope is withdrawn and the IUD is removed with grasping forceps. If this fails, a 3-mm hysteroscope with a 3.5-x-5-mm operating channel is introduced after applying a paracervical block. The IUD is then removed with endoforceps under direct vision.

In our series, the IUD was easily removed in 47 of 82 patients. The small operating hysteroscope had to be used in six of these cases.

In two patients, extraction of the IUD required general anesthesia. In one patient, the IUD was embedded in the uterine isthmus and had to be morcellated with the operative hysteroscope. This was done with general anesthesia and with arrangements for laparotomy if necessary. In 13 patients ultrasonography failed to show an IUD, and hysteroscopy also showed an empty uterine cavity. In 12 of these patients, the patient had lost the IUD vaginally without noticing it; in one patient, the IUD had traversed the myometrium and lay in the greater omentum, from which it was removed laparoscopically.

Fourteen patients were referred to us for removal of an IUD during pregnancy. The gestational ages were between 7 weeks and 10 weeks. The threads were no longer visible (Table 32).

Table 32   Hysteroscopy in patients with a "lost" IUD

Unproblematic extraction after hysteroscopic localization	47
Outpatient extraction with a small operative hysteroscope	6
Extraction with an operative hysteroscope and general anesthesia	2
Extraction with a small operative hysteroscope during pregnancy	14
Empty uterine cavity (1 patient with perforation into the abdomen)	13
Total	82

In all these cases, the IUD was first located by ultrasound (Figs. 127—129). Thus, the hysteroscopist knows preoperatively where to direct the scope and can estimate the risk for the pregnancy. The risk for the pregnancy is higher if the IUD is in the chorionic plate than if it is in the opposite decidua (Fig. 130).

Preoperatively, the patient is informed that the IUD extraction can damage the amniotic sac, in which case curettage would be necessary. The extraction is thus carried out with preparations for general anesthesia. The procedure itself requires no analgesia since the small operative hysteroscope is easily introduced into the uterine cavity during pregnancy. The cavity is dilated with physiologic saline. This is simply a safety precaution since it is not known whether diffusion of CO_2 might not cause a toxic reaction of the fetus. In contrast, Lindemann (1989), considers CO_2 the ideal medium for dilation, also during pregnancy. But since the pregnant uterus is easily distended, CO_2 flow should not exceed 20 mL/minute.

After the cervical canal has been passed, the amnion and the decidua appear (Fig. **129**). The threads of the IUD usually lie free in the uterus; the IUD itself can be hidden in the decidua (Fig. **130**). The threads of the IUD or the IUD itself is grasped with the small endoscopic forceps and withdrawn together with the hysteroscope.

Ultrasound is repeated directly after the procedure and usually still shows saline solution in the uterine cavity (Fig. **131**), which is absorbed in a few hours (Fig. **132**). The patient is usually observed in the hospital for one day and then discharged after a final ultrasound study. This procedure has been successful in all patients who desired removal of the IUD with preservation of the pregnancy.

In summary, outpatient hysteroscopy is the method of choice for retrieving a "lost" IUD. It is usually easily performed (Hepp 1977, Valle et al. 1977, Wagner 1980). If, after hysteroscopic localization, the IUD cannot be easily removed with an instrument such as grasping forceps, the examination should be repeated with a small-caliber operative hysteroscope after a paracervical block. This is almost always successful. If the patient wishes to leave an appropriately located IUD with dislocated threads in place, the threads can simply be pulled back down through the

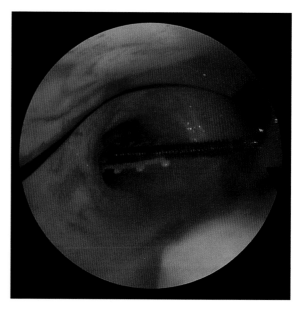

Fig. **126**   Hysteroscopic view of a dislocated IUD in the uterus

cervical canal after penetration of the myometrium has been ruled out. An IUD that has become embedded in the uterine wall can be removed with an operative hysteroscope and general anesthesia. In this case, the patient should be informed that laparoscopy or laparotomy may become necessary.

A new approach to preventing ascending infection, one of the main complications of IUD (Neis et al. 1982), is the "threadless" IUD. This is a regular IUD with the threads cut off before insertion. These IUDs can be inserted and removed only by hysteroscopy.

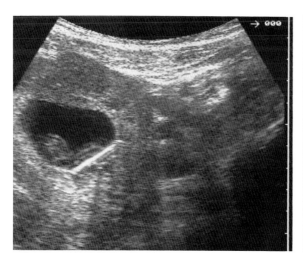 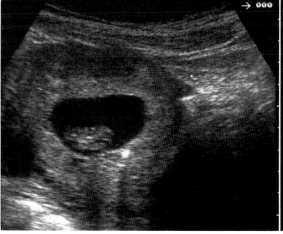

Figs. **127, 128**   Ultrasonographic images of an intact pregnancy at 10 weeks gestation with an IUD to the left of the decidua

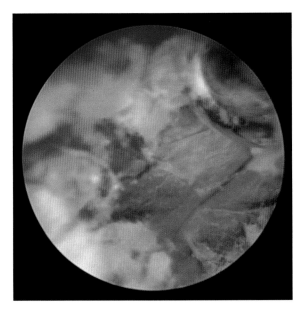

Fig. **129**   Hysteroscopic view of the amniotic epithelium at 11 weeks' gestation

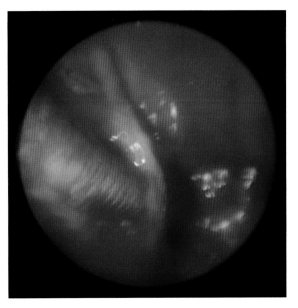

Fig. **130**   Hysteroscopy at 11 weeks' gestation shows an IUD deep in the decidua

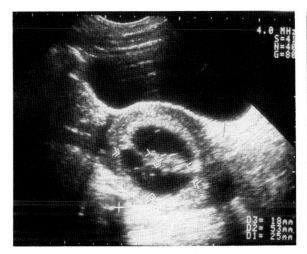

Fig. **131**   Residual dilation medium (physiologic saline) after hysteroscopic IUD extraction

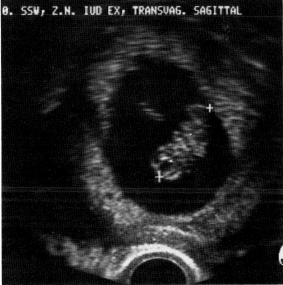

Fig. **132**   Transvaginal ultrasonography 8 hours after hysteroscopic IUD retrieval shows an intact pregnancy and no more dilation medium (same patient as in Figs. **127, 128** and **131**)

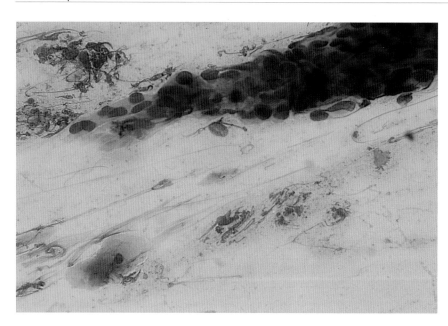

Fig. **133**   Cytologic smear from the endocervix evaluated as PAP III. The differential diagnosis includes marked cervical cell hyperplasia and endometrial hyperplasia

Unclear Cervical Smears

Unclear cytologic findings—i. e., all cervical smears classified as Papanicolaou III to V—without colposcopic correlates are indications for hysteroscopy. Careful inspection of the cervical canal and the uterine cavity can reveal or exclude a malignant lesion. This applies to endometrial conditions, 60% of which cause cytologic abnormalities (Neis et al. 1984) (Fig. **133**), as well as to adenocarcinomas and squamous cell carcinomas of the cervix with targeted streak curettage for intrauterine tissue and complete cervical curettage for intracervical tissue.

Targeted intracervical biopsies, which in our experience yield little information, are made superfluous by this procedure. It is simple and almost always provides a definitive diagnosis, even when cytologic findings are unclear.

The results are either an indication for further surgical measures (e. g., conization or hysterectomy), or they rule out neoplasia.

Other Indications

A number of hysteroscopies are performed for uncommon indications or for research purposes outside routine clinical practice. In endometrial diagnostics, research topics have included the effects of treatment for endometriosis, the effects of GnRH analogues or tamoxifen in breast cancer patients, the preoperative exclusion of endometrial carcinoma in patients with leiomyomas and menometrorrhagia, the condition of the endometrium in older patients after long-term use of oral contraceptives, and the exclusion of a placental polyp 6 weeks postpartum in a patient with a "probably" complete placenta.

We have also performed hysteroscopy in occasional patients with pelvic tumors in whom the results of palpation, ultrasound, and computed tomography

were unclear as to whether the tumor originated from the uterus or from the adnexa. One such patient had a metastasis of an ovarian carcinoma in the uterine isthmus.

A further infrequent indication for hysteroscopy is a history of contact bleeding without a colposcopic or cytologic correlate in patients in whom an intrauterine cause of bleeding was to be ruled out. One such patient showed a small squamous cell carcinoma high in the endocervix.

We have also performed outpatient hysteroscopies in patients with metastases of an unknown primary tumor whose morphology raised the suspicion of endometrial or cervical carcinoma. In most cases, hysteroscopy clarified the clinical or scientific question by revealing or ruling out a lesion of the uterus.

Thus, for experienced operators, hysteroscopy has a spectrum of possible applications beyond the classic indications (Siegler & Valle 1988, Valle 1988, Wheeler & DeCherney 1988).

Investigation of Infertility and Sterility

It is sometimes not clear whether the uterine findings in a particular patient are the actual cause of impaired fertilization, implantation, or completion of pregnancy.

Similar variations in different patients do not necessarily lead to the same functional disturbances. Infertility and sterility can have multiple causes, and it is often difficult to evaluate the role of a uterine variant. A complete assessment, including andrologic studies of the male, is necessary before the decision for surgery is made.

Intrauterine causes of sterility and infertility can be congenital (malformations) or acquired (myomas, polyps, and adhesions).

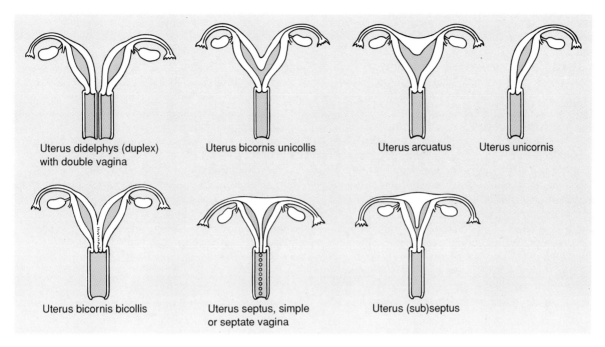

Fig. **134**   Schematic representation of the most important malformations of the female genital tract

Uterine Malformations

Uterine malformations result from inhibition of the normal fusion of the müllerian ducts. Developmentally, they fuse first in the area of the vagina and then up to the uterine fundus. Fusion can halt at various stages, with the resulting malformations. Thus, duplication of the vagina is always associated with duplication of the uterus, whereas patients with a septate or subseptate uterus may have a single vagina.

The most important malformations of the uterus and vagina are shown in Fig. **134**.

Malformations of the müllerian duct organs occur in around 5% of all women. However, only 20% of these patients have fertility problems requiring treatment. Fertilization and implantation are usually normal, but problems can arise as the pregnancy progresses. Implantation in the poorly vascularized tissue of a uterine septum can result in early spontaneous abortion. As the uterus grows, its ability to distend may be impaired, leading to premature labor. Daly et al. (1989) reported that patients with a history of miscarriage in the second trimester or premature labor in the last trimester benefited little from resection of a uterine septum. Such an operation was most likely to help patients with a history of first trimester spontaneous abortion.

The severity of a müllerian malformation is not directly related to the disturbance of fertility. Thus, 80% of pregnancies in women with a double uterus are free of complications (Berle 1985).

Diagnosis of Uterine Malformations

The large majority of uterine and vaginal malformations remain asymptomatic for a long time. An abnormality may be detected at a gynecologic examination, for instance within the framework of contraceptive counseling. Occasionally, a vaginal septum is an impediment to intercourse.

If examination shows a double vagina or high vaginal septum and two cervices, the diagnosis of uterus duplex (didelphys) is clear.

Intrauterine malformations with only one cervix (i. e., bicornate uterus or septate uterus) are usually not detected if the findings at bimanual examination are normal. If a malformation is suspected, ultrasound can often provide more information, particularly transvaginally (Perino et al. 1987). Nonetheless, hysteroscopy should always be carried out in such patients to directly visualize the uterine cavity and the extent of the malformation. Hysteroscopy either rules out a malformation or describes it (Fayez et al. 1987, La Sala et al. 1987, Sorensen 1987, Wiswedel 1987, Fedele et al. 1988, Mencaglia et al. 1988, Pellicier 1988).

The hysteroscopic description of the anatomical condition of the uterine cavity is usually straightforward. The procedure should be performed in the early proliferative phase when the endometrium is only slightly built up, thus permitting the best evaluation of the anatomy. It is advisable to first advance the hysteroscope only as far as the isthmus for a panoramic view. If the hysteroscope is too close to the fundus, a normal uterus can be mistaken for a malformation such as an arcuate uterus.

Hysteroscopy alone cannot distinguish with certainty between a septate and a bicornate uterus. If the wall between the two uterine cavities is thin, and if both tubal ostia can be seen simultaneously from the isthmus, a septum is very likely. If the tubal ostia are far apart, and if they can be visualized only by advancing the hysteroscope further into the uterus, it is likely that there are two separate uterine bodies.

Hysterosalpingography usually provides little additional information on the nature of the malformation. But particularly for the beginner, it has the advantage of confirming the diagnosis. If an operation is planned, the uterine abnormality can be measured on a hysterosalpingogram. Also, in occasional patients, information about tubal function may be desired.

A definitive diagnosis requires laparoscopy to differentiate between a septate or arcuate uterus and a bicornate uterus. This is relevant because the surgical management of these conditions differs. It is advisable to perform laparoscopy at the same session as hysteroscopy. If laparoscopy shows an externally normal uterus, the uterine septum can be removed hysteroscopically; if there are two uterine horns, an abdominal operation is necessary.

Acquired Conditions

Among the acquired causes of sterility, intrauterine adhesions (synechiae) are a special group in that they are nearly exclusively iatrogenic. In the medical histories of 258 such patients, Sugimoto et al. (1984) found 252 curettages postpartum or postabortum; 83 of the patients had had a postoperative infection. Of the remaining patients, seven had undergone enucleation of a leiomyoma, eight had undergone cesarean section, and only one had had a diagnostic curettage.

The clinical and histopathologic features of this condition were described first by Fritsch (1884) and later by Veit, Halban, and Strassmann. In 1948 Asherman pointed out the clinical significance of the syndrome, which came to bear his name. The clinical picture of Asherman syndrome includes amenorrhea, hypomenorrhea, and dysmenorrhea. Fertility is impaired by early spontaneous abortion, repeated abortion, premature delivery, and disorders of placental separation (Foix et al. 1966).

Intrauterine adhesions result from the vulnerability of the endometrium during pregnancy. Vigorous curettage can remove not only the placenta and the decidua, but also the basal membrane, leaving only the "naked" myometrium. If two such areas are opposed to each other, conglutinations can develop between them. Sugimoto distinguished three degrees of adhesions:

- Slight adhesions. These are thin and translucent and consist only of endometrium (Figs. **135, 136**)
- Moderate adhesions. These are relatively plump and the surface is covered by endometrium (Fig. **137**)
- Severe adhesions. These are also thick and plump but consist only of connective tissue

Wamstecker (1989) developed an expanded classification including the severity of the synechiae and other criteria (Table **33**). Since the location and extent of the adhesions determine the preoperative symptoms and the prognosis, this classification has been accepted by most European hysteroscopists. Thus, 81.3% of patients after lysis of slight adhesions were able to carry a pregnancy to term compared to 31.9% of patients with severe adhesions (Valle & Sciarra 1988).

Endometrial polyps have often been suspected of hindering fertilization and implantation, particularly when located near the tubal ostia. However, endometrial polyps are very rare in premenopausal women. Such findings are probably often mucosal folds that look like polyps because of magnification and distortion if the optics are brought very close to the endometrium.

In 143 patients with a diagnosis of endometrial polyps (n = 9) or "polypous lesions" (n = 134), Lübke (1984) was unable to confirm the diagnosis histologically in 138 patients. Lindemann (1988) considers such findings to represent no hindrance to fertilization because they are shed at the next menstruation. Accordingly, a lesion should be documented as persisting after menstruation before being diagnosed as a functional polyp.

How large must a true polyp be to cause sterility or infertility? The same question applies to submucosal myomas, which may prevent implantation in a way similar to an IUD. In the work-up of patients before in vitro fertilization, Bardt et al. (1987) left small leiomyomas and polyps in place because they assumed that they were not a hindrance for implantation or for a subsequent pregnancy (Fig. **138**).

In contrast, larger leiomyomas can cause miscarriages in almost 20% of patients (Robins 1982).

Table **33** Classification of the Asherman syndrome (Wamsteker 1989)

I.	Thin, delicate adhesions – Easily divided with the shaft of the hysteroscope – Tubal angles normal
II.	Isolated solid adhesions – In various areas of the cavity – Both tubal ostia visible – Not divisible with the shaft of the hysteroscope
II.a	Stenosing adhesions only in the area of the internal os – Upper uterine cavity normal
III.	Multiple solid adhesions – In various areas of the cavity – One tubal angle closed
III.a	Extensive scarring of the uterine cavity – With amenorrhea or marked hypomenorrhea
III.b	Combination of III and III.a
IV.	Extensive solid adhesions with fusion of the anterior and posterior uterine walls – Both tubal angles closed

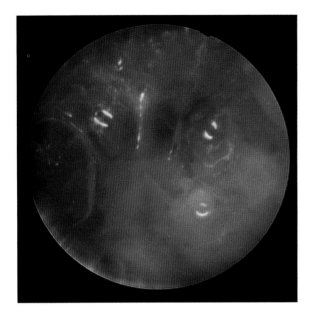

Fig. **135**   View toward the uterine fundus shows delicate synechiae

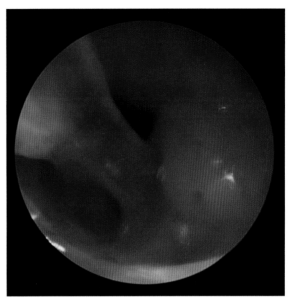

Fig. **136**   Delicate synechiae as seen with higher magnification. These adhesions are easily divided with the hysteroscope

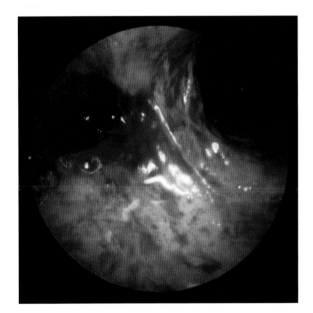

Fig. **137**   Broad, plump synechiae of connective tissue covered with endometrium. These adhesions cannot be divided with the hysteroscope only

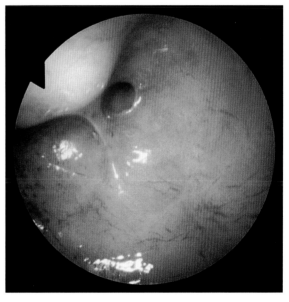

Fig. **138**   Tubal ostia in the early proliferative phase with adjacent submucosal leiomyoma. It is unclear whether this leiomyoma was the cause of the patient's sterility

Nearly half of previously infertile patients carry pregnancies to term after leiomyoma enucleation (Babaknia 1978).

Hysterosalpingography showes such lesions in 5% to 8% of sterile or infertile patients, while hysteroscopy reveales a possible uterine cause of sterility or infertility in almost 25% of patients. However, this does not mean that hysteroscopy is superior to hysterosalpingography, because the large majority of hysteroscopic diagnoses were endometrial polyps.

Taylor et al. (1987) performed hysteroscopy in 227 patients with infertility or sterility. The rate of abnormalities when CO_2 was used to distend the uterine cavity was only 25% of that when dextran was used. The authors concluded that technical artifacts are sometimes interpreted as uterine or endometrial abnormalities.

Nonetheless, hysteroscopy should be performed before embarking on any invasive therapy for sterility or infertility, particularly before in vitro fertilization and embryo transfer (Seinera et al. 1988).

Hysteroscopy permits a limited assessment of the patency of the tubes. If the intrauterine pressure is slowly increased via the hysteroflator, CO_2 escapes through the tubal ostia if the tubes are open. One sees either contractions of the ostia or bubbles on their way out of the cavity (Figs. **139, 140**).

Because it is often hard to judge the exact role of a particular finding in causing sterility and infertility, we find it useful to distinguish between possible and probable causes of infertility (Table **34**). Whereas large leiomyomas or extensive adhesions are probable causes and therefore should be treated early, this is not necessarily the case with small leiomyomas, limited adhesions, and polyps. The latter

patients can first be treated expectantly. A wait-and-see approach is also appropriate initially for patients with uterine malformations since only 20% of these impair fertility. This is important to remember because the risks connected with surgery increase with the extent of operations such as Strassman metroplasty.

Table **34**   Causes of infertility

Possible causes	Probable causes
Uterine malformations	Large leiomyomas
Small leiomyomas	Extensive, severe adhesions
Limited, slight adhesions	
Polyps	

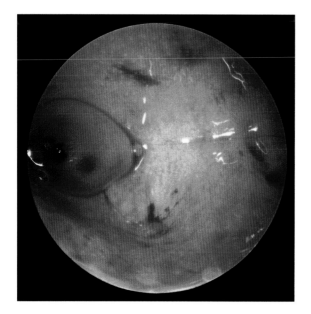 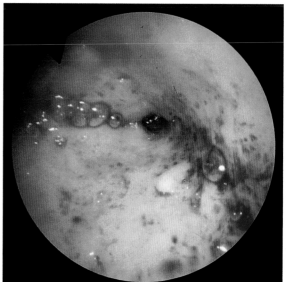

Figs. **139** and **140** CO_2 bubbles escaping through the tubal ostia

Operative Hysteroscopy

An increasing proportion of hysteroscopies is being done for surgical purposes. The steady advance of intrauterine surgery has been driven by two factors. First, in addition to simple mechanical instruments, a wide range of sophisticated laser and electrosurgical tools that can be used for a wide range of indications is available today. Second, in the age of minimally invasive surgery, the traditional indications for hysterectomy are being reevaluated critically. Both the improvements in hysteroscopic techniques and technology and the increasing desire of many patients to preserve their bodily integrity are advancing the cause of operative hysteroscopy. The method would become even more attractive if transuterine sterilization could be performed with the same safety and reliability as laparoscopic tubal sterilization.

Instruments

Operative Hysteroscopes

The thin shaft of a diagnostic hysteroscope contains only the telescope and a narrow channel for the distension medium. In contrast, the shaft of an operative hysteroscope contains the optical system, afferent and efferent channels for the distension medium, and a channel for instruments and laser fibers that can be manipulated with an Albarran mechanism or for cutting loops and other electrodes (Fig. **141**). Nonetheless, most operative hysteroscopes are only 7 mm to 8 mm in diameter. The most commonly used telescopes are 4 mm in diameter and have an optical angle of 12° (in contrast to the 25° to 30° angles of diagnostic hysteroscopes). A 12° angle is the most practicable for following the surgical instrument for the largest part of its excursion.

Surgical Instruments

A variety of biopsy forceps, grasping forceps, scissors, and special IUD forceps are available. The instruments are advanced into the uterus through the operative channel of the hysteroscope, where they are applied

Fig. **141** Operative hysteroscope

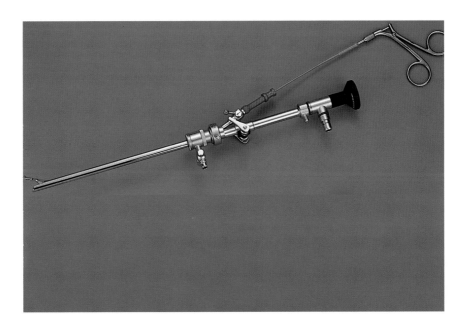

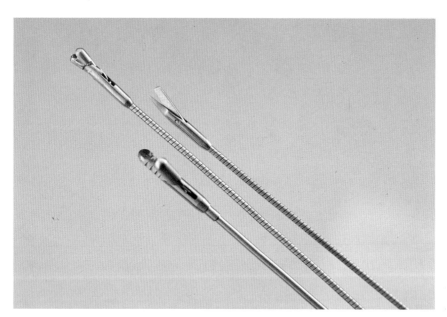

Fig. **142**   Flexible instruments

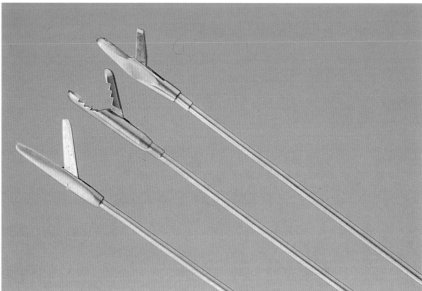

Fig. **143**   Semiflexible instruments

under direct vision (Fig. **141**). These instruments have to be flexible because they are introduced into the operative channel of the hysteroscope from below. This and their 2-mm diameter makes them fragile and easily damaged. They have to be handled with care during the procedure and during cleaning (Figs. **142, 143**). As an alternative to flexible instruments, markedly more robust semiflexible instruments and forceps and scissors integrated into the working channel of the hysteroscope have been developed (Fig. **144**).

Mechanical instruments are still widely used to retrieve IUDs and obtain biopsies, but laser and electrosurgical techniques are often preferred for dividing or resecting tissue because they obtain better hemostasis.

Laser Fibers

Lasers were used early on in the evolution of operative hysteroscopy (Goldrath et al. 1981). The considerable amount of smoke produced by laser applications requires a continuous flow of CO_2 or a liquid medium through the uterine cavity. The Nd:YAG laser is the most common type of laser system used for operative hysteroscopy. Argon lasers and particularly CO_2 lasers penetrate tissue inadequately, and a flexible fiber system for the latter is not available (Wallwiener et al. 1993).

The Nd:YAG laser is usually applied with a bare quartz fiber (Fig. **145**). The bare fiber is flexible enough to be maneuverable in the uterus and is comparatively inexpensive. If the tip is broken, the fiber simply has to be shortened. Sapphire tips are

Fig. **144**   Rigid instruments integrated into the hysteroscope shaft

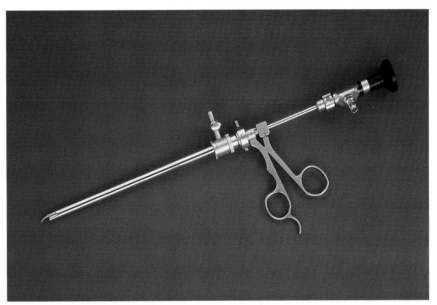

Fig. **145**   Laser fiber that can be directed with a ramp

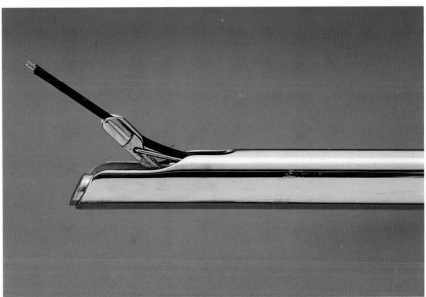

obsolete for hysteroscopy. At fluid hysteroscopy sapphire tips are cooled by the distension medium (Loffer 1990); at CO_2 hysteroscopy, they require an additional gas flow of 500 mL/minute to 800 mL/minute through the uterine cavity. This coaxial gas cooling has caused severe complications including operative deaths (Baggish & Caniell 1989, ECRI 1989, Schroeder et al. 1989), which for a time, hurt the reputation of laser hysteroscopy.

Resectoscopes

In urology, resectoscopes have long been used for transurethral resection of prostatic adenomas and for removing papillomas of the bladder. Modifying these instruments for operative hysteroscopy was a logical step (Fig. **146**).

With a pistol-like grip, a spring-loaded mechanism is used to axially advance and retract cutting loops, roller balls (cylinders), or needle electrodes of different sizes over the surgical field under direct vision. The electric current is turned on and off with a foot pedal (Fig. **147**). The best power setting for resection is just under that necessary to create a light arc, a phenomenon that in turn depends on the resistance of the tissue and the momentary area of contact between the electrode and the surgical field. Modern high-frequency electrical generators automatically adapt their output to the resistance of the tissue.

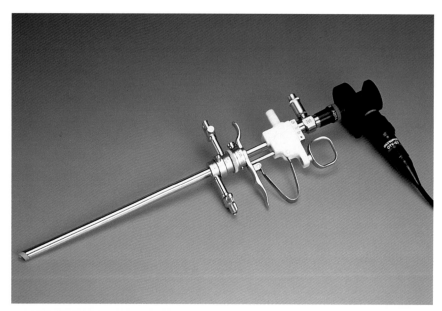

Fig. **146**   Resectoscope with video camera

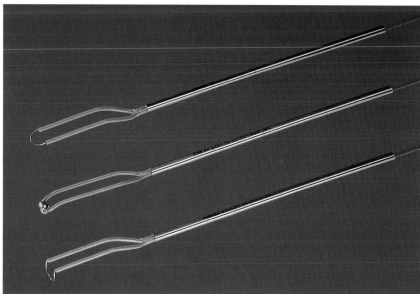

Fig. **147**   Instruments for endometrial resection and coagulation

Medical Preparation for Operative Hysteroscopy

The majority of operative hysteroscopies are performed for intrauterine conditions in patients with infertility or refractory uterine bleeding. Transuterine tubal sterilization is a further indication for selected patients.

Because the overview of the uterine cavity is much better when the endometrium is low, hysteroscopic operations are best performed during the early proliferative phase of the menstrual cycle—i. e., soon after menstrual bleeding has stopped. A high endometrium, as during the secretory phase of the cycle, obscures vision.

It is very helpful to treat patients medically before ablating or resecting the endometrium or myomas. The goal is to induce atrophy of the endometrium,

which makes the operation easier and reduces the incidence of renewed abnormal vaginal bleeding. Typical regimens are two cycles of a gonadotropin-releasing hormone (GnRH) analogue such as goserelin or leuproreline acetate, a low-dose progestin (e. g., lynestrenol 15 mg/day, dydrogesterone 20 mg/day for 4 to 6 weeks), or danazol (400-600 mg/day) for 6 weeks before surgery. Low-dose progestin treatment is less expensive than the other regimens but may not be as effective.

We also pretreat patients scheduled for myoma resection. Treatment with a GnRH analogue for 3 months caused myomas to shrink by an average of 38%, with some disappearing completely. However, in almost half the patients, the size of the myomas is unaffected by medical treatment (Healy et al. 1984, Donnez et al. 1989, Van der Spruy et al. 1989, Hackenberg et al. 1990, Donnez et al. 1990, Gresenhues et al. 1990, Gallinat 1992).

Apart from these endocrine measures, the blood supply to the surgical field can be reduced temporarily by paracervical infiltration with vasopressin at surgery (Valle et al. 1991).

Infertility and Sterility

Both of these conditions can have uterine causes, and diagnostic hysteroscopy is indicated if such a cause is suspected. To obtain the best view, hysteroscopy should be performed in the early proliferative phase of the menstrual cycle—i. e., soon after menstruation, when the endometrium is lowest. Uterine causes of sterility can be congenital (uterine malformations), acquired (polyps and myomas), or iatrogenic (synechiae, Asherman's syndrome). Even though such lesions cannot be proved to cause infertility, if they are present the patient should be advised to undergo operative hysteroscopy to treat them. It is likely that such lesions can hinder implantation and nidation (similar to the mechanism of an IUD) or affect the blood supply to the conceptus after implantation. A survey by the American Association of Gynecological Laparoscopists in 1988 found fertility disorders to be the second most common indication for operative hysteroscopy (27% of procedures) (Peterson et al. 1990). Surgical interventions in patients with infertility should be performed in conjunction with measures addressing other problems (endocrine disorders, tubal conditions, andrologic factors) as indicated.

Polyps and Myomas

Endometrial polyps are uncommon in patients being evaluated for infertility (Toro-Calzada et al. 1992). Nonetheless, if found, an intrauterine polyp should be removed to obtain a specimen for histology and to avoid, or to treat, dysfunctional uterine bleeding. In practice this usually means locating a polyp by hysteroscopy and then removing it by careful curettage. Hysteroscopy should be repeated after curettage to determine whether the polyp has been removed completely. If not, the base of a polyp can be divided with hysteroscopic scissors, a laser, or a resectoscope. To avoid recurrence, care should be taken to resect or eradicate the entire base of the polyp.

Myomas can cause infertility by altering the endometrial vascularization and disturbing the conditions for nidation of the conceptus (Fig. **148**) (Babaknia et al. 1978). Like polyps, myomas are seen much more commonly in patients being evaluated for dysfunctional bleeding than in those with infertility. The procedure for resecting myomas is thus discussed in the section on dysfunctional uterine bleeding. All patients receive hormonal treatment before the operation to achieve endometrial atrophy. Atrophy improves the overview of the uterine cavity, thus often revealing further myomas (Vancaillie 1988). It can also shrink myomas and reduce the blood supply to the surgical field.

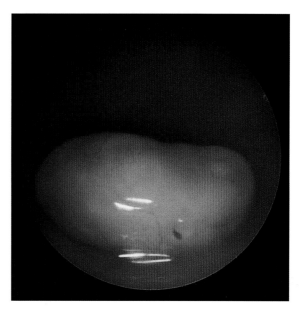

Fig. **148**   Solitary, completely intracavitary myoma

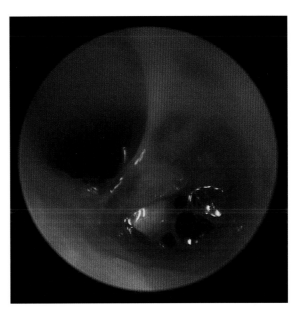

Fig. **149**   Endometrial bridges. These can be mistaken for synechiae or a septum

Synechiae

Intrauterine synechiae in a patient with infertility or sterility always represent an indication for endoscopic lysis because they can be considered to hinder nidation and to cause early spontaneous abortion (Fig. **149**). According to Hamou (1981), intrauterine adhesions are classified as endometrial, myofibrous, or fibrous.

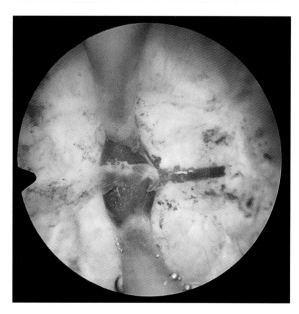

Fig. **150**   Lysis of severe intrauterine adhesions with a needle electrode

Synechiae are diagnosed at hysteroscopy in the early proliferative phase. This improves visibility and ensures that endometrial synechiae (grade 1 lesions), which in our experience are most common in the secretory phase, are not mistaken for more advanced conditions. Purely endometrial bridges surely do not hinder implantation of the conceptus or expansion of the uterine cavity later in pregnancy. Because we have seen such lesions even in patients with primary sterility without previous curettage, we suspect that they are merely endometrial adhesions between the anterior and posterior uterine walls arising from the artificial distension of the uterine cavity. The increased mucous content of the endometrium in the second half of the cycle may also explain why these bridges, which we call pseudosynechiae, are seen most commonly during this phase. Typically, they are lysed by merely touching them with the hysteroscope—further evidence that they are simple bridges of the endometrium rather than structural lesions.

Sugimoto et al. (1984) reported on 258 patients with intrauterine adhesions. Adequate reduction of adhesions was achieved in 246 patients (71 with grade 1 synechiae) with the hysteroscope shaft alone or, in difficult cases, by opening the hysteroscopic forceps in the uterine cavity. Surprisingly, all 34 patients with amenorrhea preoperatively developed a regular menstrual cycle after the procedure. Of the 258 patients, 107 later became pregnant. Hamou (1983), Taylor & Hamou (1982), Levin & Neuwirth (1973), and March et al. (1987) have reported similar results. Other authors (Valle & Sciarra 1984, Vancaillie 1988) prefer small endoscopic scissors. While less severe adhesions can be reduced by simply distending the uterine cavity or with endoscissors, extensive intrauterine adhesions, as in patients with full-blown Asherman's syndrome, require careful division of the tissue with a laser or needle electrode (Fig. **150**).

Intraoperative perforation of the uterus is uncommon if the synechiae are mild, but the uterine wall can be thin if there is a history of uterine surgery. Simultaneous laparoscopy should be performed in these patients to avoid perforation and is also advisable if the extent of the intrauterine adhesions leads the operator to suspect occlusion of the tubes or if tubal occlusion has been diagnosed previously by hysterosalpingography. Chromopertubation through the hysteroscope shaft should be performed at the end of the adhesiolysis to confirm a satisfactory result.

Almost all authors place an IUD or a Foley catheter into the uterine cavity after adhesiolysis to prevent renewed adhesion of the uterine walls. The Foley catheter also ensures hemostasis and is left in place for 1 or 2 days; an IUD can be left in place longer.

Adjuvant hormonal treatment is controversial (Vercellini et al. 1989) because endogenous hormone production in young women should be sufficient to adequately stimulate the remaining endometrium. March & Israel (1981, 1987) administered 2.5 mg of estradiol per day for 60 days and obtained a pregnancy rate of almost 90% and a spontaneous abortion rate of only 7.5%. These results, which are markedly better than those reported by other authors, may be due to the technique of carefully reducing even the smallest adhesions with scissors. Vancaillie (1988) considers estrogen administration necessary only after the reduction of grade 3 to grade 4 lesions according to Wamsteker.

In our experience, hysteroscopic lysis of intrauterine adhesions is rarely possible during outpatient diagnostic hysteroscopy. Outpatient hysteroscopic lysis makes sense only if the uterine cavity can easily be dilated with the shaft under direct vision step-by-step and if a completely open cavity is the result. If not, the adhesions should be reduced with a laser or resectoscope to produce the least trauma. The decision to perform laparoscopy is made during the procedure. The surgeon should know that perforation of the uterus is a typical complication and that cases of spontaneous uterine rupture during subsequent pregnancies have been reported and are probably due to an abnormally thin uterine wall (Deaton et al. 1989).

Hysteroscopic reduction of synechiae is thus performed only if anesthesia can be induced if necessary. If the patient reports pain during adhesiolysis or if laparoscopy becomes necessary, the intrauterine operation should be interrupted until anesthesia has been induced.

Like Vercellini et al. (1989) and Assaf et al. (1990), who take no adjuvant measures after surgery and report adhesion-free healing of the wound surface after transcervical procedures, we no longer insert an IUD after adhesiolysis. We believe that hormonal treatment makes sense for patients in whom thick adhesions were reduced, whether on an outpatient or inpatient basis. We prescribe 1.25 mg of estradiol for 30 days followed by 10 days of 10-20 mg progesterone.

We recommend follow-up hysteroscopy, with renewed adhesiolysis if necessary, after withdrawal bleeding.

Resection of Septa

Fusion and inhibition misdevelopments of the müllerian ducts can cause a wide spectrum of conditions including mild arcuate uterus, septate uterus, duplication of the uterus and vagina, and agenesis of the müllerian ducts. The most common anomaly (80%) is partial or complete septation of the uterus (Fayez 1986). Even though some patients with these conditions have uncomplicated conception and pregnancy, the work-up of infertility or sterility should include a search for such anomalies. In a series reported by DeCherney (1984), up to 5% of patients had müllerian duct anomalies.

The surgical correction of uterine malformations long consisted of open metroplasty operations as described by Strassmann, Jones, and Tompkins. While these procedures have been reported to lead to a 75% pregnancy rate as compared with 4% in untreated patients (Wallwiener et al. 1993), they are major operations that require elective cesarean section in a subsequent pregnancy and risks of adhesions, tubal occlusion, and intraoperative bleeding. In the era of minimally invasive surgery, traditional uteroplasties should be used only if there is no alternative treatment (Khalifa et al. 1993).

Today the resection of uterine septa is in the domain of operative hysteroscopy because it is less traumatic than open metroplasty and because vaginal delivery in subsequent pregnancies is possible (Valle et al. 1991, Donnez et al. 1992). Three endoscopic techniques have been used: bipolar coagulation and subsequent division with endoscissors (March & Israel 1987, Assaf et al. 1990), resection with the Nd:YAG laser (Campo et al. 1990, Choe & Baggish 1992), and resection with the resectoscope. These techniques seem to have similar rates of success and complications. Eighty percent to 90% of subsequent pregnancies are carried to term, and intraoperative uterine perforation and postoperative synechiae are rare.

A malformation of the uterus is often first suspected at vaginal ultrasonography. If the diagnosis is confirmed at outpatient hysteroscopy, we recommend a preoperative hysterosalpingogram to obtain preoperative information on the patency of the tubes and on the width of the septum. This helps plan the operation and is important for discussing it and possible complications with the patient beforehand (Figs. **151, 152**).

Diagnostic laparoscopy is performed during the same anesthesia as the hysteroscopic operation to decide whether hysteroscopic resection of the septum is possible or whether laparotomy and metroplasty have to be performed, for example for bicornate uterus. If a uterine septum is confirmed, it is resected with an assistant watching for uterine perforation through the laparoscope.

We now prefer to resect the septum with a needle electrode because the success rates of the techniques

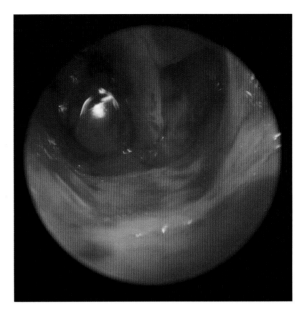

Fig. **151**   Fibrous uterine septum

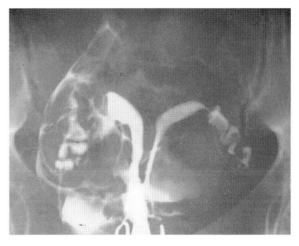

Fig. **152**   Hysterosalpingogram in the same patient as in Fig. 151

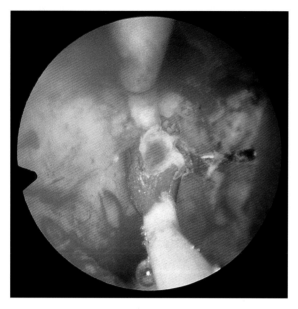

Fig. **153** Hysteroscopic reduction of a wide septum using a needle electrode

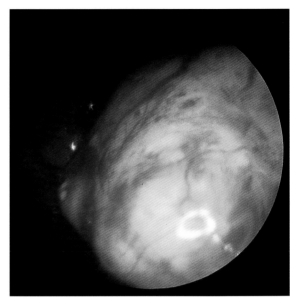

Fig. **154** Large, submucous myoma protruding into the uterine cavity

are similar and because needle resection is quicker than the conventional mechanical and the laser procedures (Fig. **153**). If follow-up hysteroscopy at 4-6 weeks shows no residual septum requiring a second procedure, we advise the patient that she is free to conceive 8 weeks after the operation.

Uterine Bleeding Disorders

Menometrorrhagia can be caused by uterine myomas at all ages of life. Other factors that can cause recurrent uterine bleeding, which is exacerbated in the presence of myomas, include endocrine dysregulation, such as follicular persistence in women approaching menopause. Systemic factors adversely affecting coagulation can also cause abnormal bleeding. Such hemorrhagic diatheses can be congenital (e. g., hemophilia), acquired (e. g., hepatic cirrhosis), or iatrogenic (e. g., anticoagulation with coumarin derivatives). Malignancy has to be ruled out (for example by outpatient hysteroscopy with streak curettage) before any treatment that includes preservation of the uterus.

Myomas, abnormal uterine bleeding, or both have long been the most common indication for hysterectomy. Today the technical advances in minimally invasive surgery and the increasing experience of a growing number of operators often make it possible to preserve the uterus. Also, this wish is expressed increasingly by patients. In a 1988 survey by the American Association of Gynecological Laparoscopists, uterine bleeding disorders were the most common indication (57%) for operative hysteroscopy (Peterson et al. 1990).

Resection of Myomas

Hysteroscopic surgery for myomas should always be preceded by a 2-3 month course of a GnRH analogue. Operative treatment is planned according to the results of vaginal ultrasonography and diagnostic hysteroscopy. The number and diameters of the myomas to be removed and their intramural component influence the surgical technique and what results the patient can be told to expect (Wamsteker et al. 1993). Largely intracavitary myomas with narrow bases are markedly easier to resect than mostly intramural myomas. A measure that describes the situation is the angle between the surface of the myoma and the adjacent myometrium. The more acute this angle, the more intracavitary the myoma (Pace et al. 1992).

Because simply dividing a narrow base of a pedunculated myoma with a snip of the scissors is rarely possible, Nd:YAG laser and high-frequency electrosurgical techniques are commonly used. The complications associated with these modalities and the steps taken to avoid them are discussed in the respective chapters.

The bare fiber of the Nd:YAG laser is used at a power of about 40 watts in CO_2 and at 80 watts or more in fluid distension media. Liquid distension media are associated with less smoke formation and provide better visibility. Dissection with the bare fiber can be done with a contact technique, which has more of a cutting effect, or with a non-touch technique, which has more of a coagulating effect (Gallinat 1992). Lasers produce less bleeding than electrosurgical techniques, but because of the limited depth of penetration, more difficult handling, and the longer

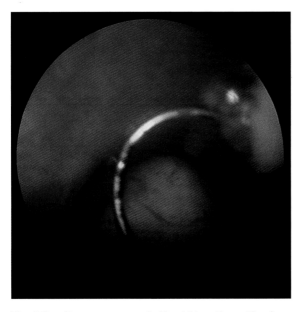

Fig. **155**   Same myoma as in Fig. 154 as the cutting loop approaches

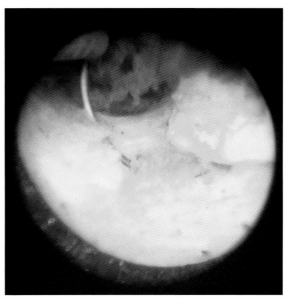

Fig. **156**   Same myoma as in Figs. 154 and 155. Piecemeal hysteroscopic resection

operating time, they are used more for treating smaller and pedunculated myomas (Campo et al. 1990, Hucke et al. 1992, Wallwiener et al. 1993).

Hysteroscopic electroresection of myomas can be performed with a needle electrode in the special case of pedunculated myomas with a narrow base. However, much more often we use a cutting loop to resect myomas in a piecemeal fashion (Figs. **154—156**). Cutting is performed at a power of 100-120 watts, coagulation at about 70 watts. Operating times are shorter than at laser surgery because the cutting loops cut better. Because even larger myomas can be resected at one sitting, the resectoscopic approach is preferred for larger and broad-based myomas (Hucke et al. 1992, Wallwiener et al. 1993). This technique permits enucleation of myomas with an intramural volume of 50% or more (Pace et al. 1992).

If a submucous myoma is located largely intramurally so that the myometrium bulges only slightly, laser coagulation and electroresection can destroy only its surface. Donnez et al. (1990) described a technique using a laser fiber or a needle electrode to puncture the myoma at one or more sites. This comparatively simple manipulation, combined with continuing endocrine therapy for another 2-3 months, often led to necrosis and subsequent resorption of the myoma.

Follow-up hysteroscopy after two cycles should be planned for all patients after myoma resection to diagnose and treat residuals. Overall, about 90% of patients achieve normal uterine bleeding patterns after hysteroscopic resection of myomas (Serden & Brooks 1991, Wamsteker et al. 1993, Indman 1993). This justifies the conservative treatment approach with

preservation of the uterus and fertility as well as the much shorter hospital stay and time away from work.

Endometrial Ablation and Resection

While isolated submucous myomas are resected hysteroscopically to preserve fertility or explicitly to treat infertility, endometrial ablation or resection aim only to treat uterine bleeding disorders while preserving the uterus. Patients undergoing resection of isolated myomas are generally younger than those undergoing endometrial resection (Brooks & Serden 1992).

After malignancy has been ruled out and the decision to preserve the uterus has been made, the endometrium should be brought into atrophy by medical treatment to improve visibility in the uterine cavity and to improve the results of surgery. The endometrium can then be eradicated with a laser in a gas or liquid medium, resected with a resectoscope, or ablated with a roller ball.

The Nd:YAG laser with a bare quartz fiber has proven useful for photocoagulating the endometrium, as for resecting myomas. At a power of 40 watts in a CO_2 milieu, the laser penetrates 4 mm to 6 mm into tissue. This suffices to coagulate atrophic endometrium with the basal lamina and may even destroy subbasal foci of adenomyosis. The endometrium is vaporized with the bare fiber in furrows, beginning in the uterine fundus and continuing toward the isthmus (Fig. **157**).

Electrosurgical ablation with a roller ball or resection with a cutting loop is performed in a fluid distension medium. Here too, the procedure is begun in the fundus and continued down to the isthmus. The 90°

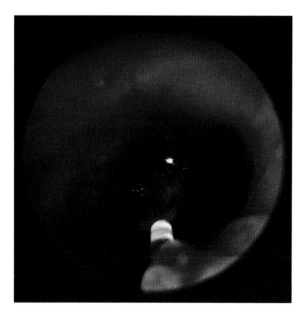

Fig. **157**   Endometrial ablation with a laser

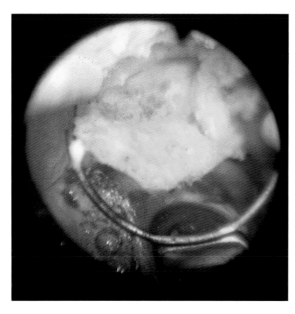

Fig. **158**   Endometrial ablation. Careful elevation of a strip of tissue from the endometrium and superficial myometrium

approach of the instrument and its axial excursion make the endometrium in the fundus difficult to resect with a cutting loop without a high risk of perforation. Thus, we coagulate the endometrium in this area with the roller ball. We also prefer the roller ball for the uterine cornua and the tubal angles, where the myometrium is thin. A number of authors perform the entire procedure with the roller ball. This is simpler technically and entails a lower risk of perforation, but care has to be taken to pass the cylinder slowly over the tissue to achieve adequate coagulation. We prefer resecting the endometrium of the anterior and posterior uterine walls with cutting loops. The endometrium is resected strip-by-strip beginning at 6 o'clock and proceeding in a clockwise direction (Fig. **158**). The depth of the resection is adjusted to the bleeding and to the depth of the preceding furrow. Increasing bleeding indicates resection down into the myometrium. At intervals, the telescope is withdrawn, and the tissue fragments in the cavity are retrieved with a curet or forceps and sent for histology.

Both laser photocoagulation and electroresection have been reported to have success rates of 80% to 94% (DeCherney et al. 1987, Magos et al. 1989, Davis 1989, Pyper & Haeri 1991, Brun et al. 1991) and were similar in a direct comparison (Petrucco & Gillespie 1991). Laser ablation has been associated with less intraoperative bleeding and a lower rate of postoperative intrauterine adhesions, which was ascribed to a more thorough coagulation of the endometrium (Gallinat 1992). Also, in a review of 4038 patients, the rate of uterine perforation was lower for laser procedures (Macdonald et al. 1992). But the longer operating times and more difficult technical execution of laser procedures have led us and most other authors to prefer electrosurgical methods for routine use.

Whatever method is used, subsequent pregnancy cannot be ruled out in patients with normal ovarian function. We thus recommend simultaneous laparoscopic tubal sterilization.

The endometrium in the uterine isthmus should be spared at resection to avoid subsequent development of mucometra or hematometra. This is important with regard to the early detection of endometrial cancer in the future, which is a small but present risk (Copperman et al. 1993). Also, patients should continue to have regular gynecologic exams after endometrial ablation or resection.

Uterine perforation occurs in 2% to 3% of procedures and is more common with inexperienced operators (Magos et al. 1991; Macdonald et al. 1992). Perforation can be avoided by careful surgery and by respecting contraindications. The operator should have extensive experience with diagnostic hysteroscopy before performing his or her first intrauterine operations under the supervision of an experienced colleague (see also "Complications of Operative Procedures"). Itzkowic & Beale (1992) reported that the risk of perforation is higher in patients who have had a cesarean section.

Before the operation, the patient should understand that complete amenorrhea is not necessarily the goal. Especially for patients with large uteri (as reflected by a long sound length), stable hypomenorrhea or eumenorrhea, which develops in 10% to 20% of patients, represents successful treatment. A less radical approach also has advantages. Brun et al. (1992) reported intrauterine adhesions in up to 70% of patients after extensive resection while Gallinat (1992), whose therapeutic goal was only hypomenorrhea, saw no synechiae in his patients. This is an advantage for the detection of endometrial cancer later in life. If hypermenorrhea persists or recurs, which occurs in 10% to 20% of patients (Pyper & Haeri 1991), endometrial resection or ablation can be repeated. Patients with persisting bleeding problems after two procedures should be advised to undergo hysterectomy. The percentage of patients with recurrent bleeding problems despite repeated hysteroscopic procedures has been reported to be between 5% and 10% (DeCherney et al. 1987, Magos et al. 1991).

Intrauterine Surgery in the Individualized Treatment of Uterine Disease

Until a few years ago, the therapeutic options for the operative treatment of bleeding disorders, myomas, or both was limited almost exclusively to vaginal and abdominal hysterectomy. Many gynecologists tried to respect their patients' wishes to preserve their bodily integrity as far as possible and preferred the more natural approach to hysterectomy, the vaginal route. But due to fundamentally different surgical schools and different levels of training, the percentage of hysterectomies performed vaginally varies widely from country to country, and even from hospital to hospital.

The technological and operative advances of minimally invasive surgery have greatly expanded the spectrum of gynecologic surgery. Treatment can now be individualized. If there is an indication for hysterectomy, and traditional vaginal hysterectomy is not possible, laparotomy can increasingly be avoided by performing a laparoscopically assisted vaginal hysterectomy. This technique has permitted us to reduce the rate of hysterectomies performed abdominally to 10% to 15%. Sixty-five to 70% of the hysterectomies performed at our department are traditional vaginal procedures; the remaining patients undergo laparoscopically assisted vaginal hysterectomy.

Before a patient is advised to undergo hysterectomy, however, it should be clear that extirpating the organ is indeed necessary to cure her condition. For example, today, even large subserous myomas can usually be removed laparoscopically, and the scope of intrauterine surgery can be individualized according to the findings, complaints, and the desire to preserve fertility.

Treatment adapted to the patient's needs and complaints is far more than a fashionable trend of the Zeitgeist. The methods of minimally invasive surgery are now firmly established, and no practicing gynecologic surgeon can ignore them. Also, growing economic, medical, and political pressures favor procedures that require only a brief hospital stay and permit a quick return to work. All these considerations favor a flexible and individualized approach to patients with uterine disease.

Transuterine Tubal Sterilization

Laparoscopic tubal sterilization is currently the method of choice for female sterilization. It is simple and has a low risk of complications. The failure rate is measured per thousand procedures. However, the procedure requires general anesthesia and rare, but typical, complications, such as injury of bowel or blood vessels, can be severe. It was thus logical to try to develop a hysteroscopic technique for tubal sterilization with paracervical blockade on an outpatient basis. A number of techniques have been tried.

Brundin (1987) implanted different plugs with barbs into the intramural segment of the tube (Fig. **159**). Erb (1984) used "formed-in-place" silicon rubber plugs, which entail instilling a silicon mixture into the tubal angles under hysteroscopic guidance (Reed & Erb 1983). The material is injected in the fluid state and then congeals within about 5 minutes (Fig. **160**). Lindemann (1973), Wamsteker (1984) and other authors introduced electrodes into the intramural segment of the tube to coagulate the tubal epithelium and achieve obliteration of the lumen.

The success rates of all these hysteroscopic methods are markedly lower than that of laparoscopic sterilization. Complete sterilization is achieved in about 80% of patients (Lindemann 1981, Brundin 1987), which means that one or both tubes remain open in 20%. All patients have to undergo follow-up hysterosalpingography. The hysteroscopic procedure can be repeated if a tube is still open, but 2% to 5% of patients still have patent tubes even after second or third attempts.

Darabi & Richart (1977) compiled complication rates in a multicenter study. Among a total of 773 sterilizations, there were seven uterine perforations and seven bowel injuries with subsequent peritonitis. One patient died of an undetected bowel perforation caused with an electroprobe.

We evaluated the Nd:YAG laser for transuterine sterilization in 105 rat uteri (Otte 1992). Obliteration rates of 100% were achieved with the bare fiber with both contact and noncontact techniques. Histology, however, showed extensive destruction of the uterine surface after contact application while the noncontact technique showed a pure coagulation effect. Thus, the latter technique, which produced similar results but with minimal tissue damage, seems more promising. An optimal effect was seen by applying the laser at a power of 40 watts for a duration of 45 ± 7 seconds at a distance of 3 mm to 5 mm from the ostium. However, we do not have clinical results.

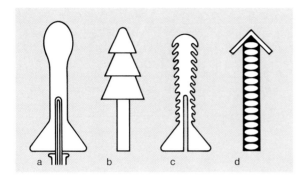

Fig. **159**   Plugs designed for insertion into the tubal ostia

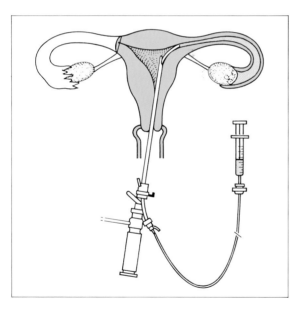

Fig. **160**   Technique for applying the formed-in-place silicon rubber plugs

Hysteroscopic sterilization is thus appropriate only for very selected patients for whom sterilization by laparoscopy or minilaparotomy is not possible. The patient has to be informed of the success and failure rates of the hysteroscopic operation, the necessity of follow-up hysterosalpingography, and that a second procedure may be necessary. This is recommended also in light of the immense damage claims made by patients who carry a pregnancy to term after attempted sterilization.

Chorionic Villus Sampling

Hysteroscopic biopsy of the chorion, suggested by Ghirardini (1985), has not been widely used. Ghirardini developed an instrument with a shaft diameter of 4 mm to obtain decidual villi between the 9th and 13th gestational weeks (Fig. **161**). The tip of the hysteroscope contains a lateral window through which chorionic villi can be aspirated. The aspirated villi are severed when the window is closed and are submitted for genetic analysis. This technique can be performed under direct vision, but the lateral window permits no straight-ahead view so that it is difficult to direct the instrument directly to the chorion frondosum (Fig. **162**).

Chorionoscopes developed by other investigators (Mencaglia et al. 1986) do not have this drawback, but it is still difficult to obtain small samples of the chorion. The instruments cannot be considered technically mature. Although the idea of chorionic villus biopsy under visual guidance is appealing, transcervical and transabdominal procedures under ultrasound guidance are simple, safe, and quickly mastered. The complication rate is low, and, at present, there is little need to replace them by an endoscopic method.

Hysteroscopic Gamete Intrafallopian Transfer

Laparoscopic gamete intrafallopian transfer (GIFT) is the method of choice to treat idiopathic and andrologic sterility (Wiedemann & Hepp 1989). In contrast to in vitro fertilization and embryo transfer (IVF & ET), GIFT entails fertilization in the physiologic milieu of the tubal ampulla. This obviates the issues of timesharing between the endometrium and the embryo that arise when the first divisions of the fertilized oocyte take place in vitro. After transvaginal follicular puncture under ultrasound guidance, IVF & ET can be performed without general anesthesia, which is not the case for GIFT.

Transuterine GIFT with a catheter would be appealing, but there have been only isolated case reports of successful hysteroscopic gamete transfers (Würfel et al. 1988). This implies that the fertilization rate lags far behind that of laparoscopic GIFT, and ethical considerations thus mitigate against hysteroscopic attempts. But hysteroscopic GIFT seems so elegant that it should be pursued further, first in animal experiments and later in careful clinical trials.

Fig. **161**   Chorionoscope

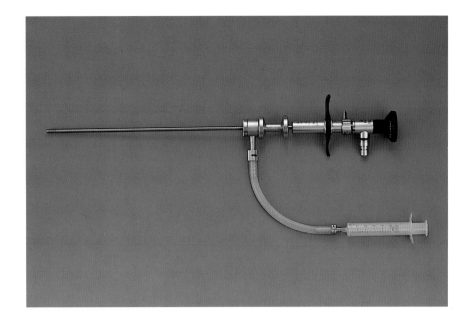

Fig. **162**   Schematic representation of chorionic villus sampling with a chorionoscope

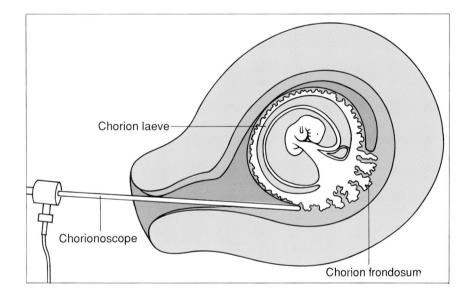

Vaginal Ultrasonography and Hysteroscopy

Endosonographic probes to visualize the bladder, rectum, and uterus have been available since the early 1980s. These high-frequency, high-resolution probes are designed to be introduced into the rectum, vagina, or other orifices and placed in the immediate vicinity of the organ to be studied. It is to the credit of Popp (1986) that transvaginal ultrasonography is now a routine procedure both in hospitals and many gynecologic offices. The technique permits immediate follow-up of unclear findings at pelvic examination. The combination of bimanual pelvic examination and vaginal ultrasonography at the same visit has a diagnostic accuracy of 95% (Sauter 1989). Vaginal ultrasonography immediately after pelvic examination involves little or no additional discomfort for the patient. Considering the high validity, low costs, and increased availability in office settings, the technique approaches the requirements of screening studies.

Vaginal ultrasonography has been evaluated in screening protocols for endometrial and ovarian cancer, diseases for which there are still no widely accepted methods for early detection. However, the effectiveness of routine ultrasonography in screening for gynecologic tumors has been questioned by Loch et al. (1984) and other authors.

Endometrial cancer, which causes symptoms early on, is usually diagnosed in stage I, in which 5-year survival rates exceed 80% (Kottmeier 1985). This will be hard to improve on by screening tests. In contrast, most ovarian cancers are still diagnosed in stage III (Neis & Branchetti 1982). This disease seems to develop so rapidly that early detection at annual examinations may not improve results.

The rapid advance of vaginal ultrasound technology in recent years has been so dramatic, however, that it seems possible to detect even minimal changes of the endometrium and ovaries. Screening protocols have to be continually reevaluated in the light of new data. Whether modified techniques, such as filling the uterine cavity (Van Roessel 1987), will increase accuracy remains to be seen.

Brandner et al. (1991) found vaginal ultrasonography to have a specificity of 94% and a sensitivity of 88% for detecting endometrial cancer. The authors were able to distinguish between atrophy, proliferated endometrium, hyperplasia, polyps, and carcinomas (Figs. **163, 168**). Sonographic evidence of hyperplasia, a polyp, or carcinoma should be pursued further. Outpatient hysteroscopy is an ideal tool in this situation.

Transvaginal ultrasonography with visualization of the uterus and ovaries after routine gynecologic examination is very attractive theoretically. Whether it will be equally convincing in practice and whether it will lead to real improvements in the rates of early detection and survival remains to be determined (Table **35**).

Table **35** Expanded screening examination of the female genital tract

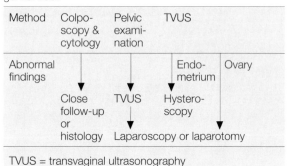

TVUS = transvaginal ultrasonography

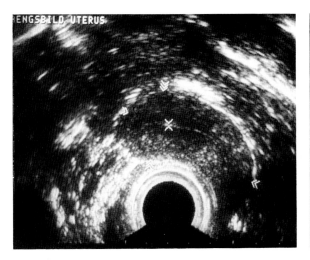

Fig. **163**   Transvaginal ultrasound scan in a patient with endometrial atrophy

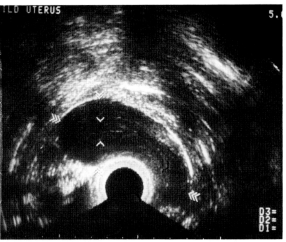

Fig. **164**   Transvaginal ultrasound scan in a patient with highly proliferated endometrium

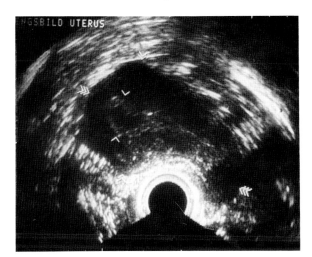

Fig. **165**   Transvaginal ultrasound scan in a patient with hyperplastic endometrium

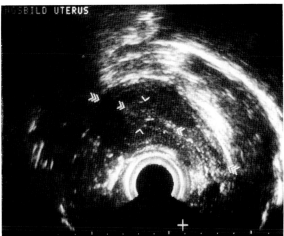

Fig. **166**   Transvaginal ultrasound scan in a patient with endometrial cancer and hematometra

References

Alvarado, D.A., G.R. Quinones: Tubal instillation of quina-crine under hysteroscopic control. In J.J. Sciarra, J.C. Beutler, J.J. Speidel: Hysteroscopic sterilization. Intercont Med. Book, New York 1974

Anastasiadis, P., M. Lüdinghausen, F. Rühl, A.M. Bowriy: Die Bedeutung der Aspirationszytologie für die Früherkennung des Korpuscarcinoms und seiner Vorstufen. Geburtsh. Frauenheilk. 41 (1981) 136

Anderson, R.K.: Electrical and thermal aspects of high-frequency electrosurgical energy as applied to hysteroscopy. In J.J. Sciarra, J.C. Butler, J.J. Speidel: Hysteroscopy Sterilization. Intercont Med. Book, New York 1984

Asherman, J.G.: Traumatic intra-uterine adhesions. J. Obstet. Gynaecol. Brit. Emp. 57 (1950) 892

Asherman, J.G.: Amenorrhea traumatica (atretrica). J. Obstet. Gynaecol. Brit. Emp. 55 (1948) 23

Assaf, A., A. El Tagy, A. El Kady, H. El Agezy: Hysteroscopic removal of copper-containing intrauterine devices with missing tails during pregnancy. Advanc. Contracept. 4 (1988) 131

Assaf A., G. Serour, A. Elkady, H. el Agizy: Endoscopic management of the intrauterine septum. Int. J. Gynecol. Obst. 32 (1990) 43

Aubinais, R.J.: Revue obstétricale-utéroscopie. L'union médicale 24 (1864) 591

Babaknia, A., J.A. Rock, Jr. H.W Jones Jr.: Pregnancy success following abdominal myomectomy for infertility. Fertil. Steril. 30 (1978) 644

Bachet, W., P. Brunner, J.D.J. Dodenhöft, E. Strobel: Diagnostische Treffsicherheit der Endometriumszytologie mit prevical. Geburtsh. Frauenheilk. 43 (1983) 11

Baggish, M.S.: Contact hysteroscopy: A new technique to explore the uterine cavity. Obstet. Gynecol. 54 (1979) 350

Baggish, M.S.: Evaluation and staging of endometrial and endocervical adenocarcinoma by contact hysteroscopy, Gynecol. Oncol. 9 (1980) 182

Baggish, M.S., J.F. Daniell: Catastrophic injury secondary to the use of coaxial gas-cooled fibers and artificial saphire tips for intrauterine surgery: A report of five cases. Lasers Surg. Med. 9 (1989) 581

Baggish, M.S., J.F. Daniell: Death caused by air embolism associated with neodymium:yttrium-aluminum-garnet laser surgery and artificial sapphire tips. Am. J. Obstet. Gynecol. 161 (1989) 877

Baggish, M.S., J.H. Dorsey: Contact hysteroscopic evaluation of the endocervix as an adjunct to colposcopy. Obstet. Gynecol. 60 (1982) 107

Baggish, M.S.: Hysteroscopic sterilization by silastic plugs. In A.M. Siegler, H.J. Lindemann: Hysteroscopy: Principles and Practice. Lippincott, Philadelphia, 1984

Baggish, M.S.: A new laser hysteroscope for neodymium-YAG endometrial ablation. Lasers Surg. Med. 8 (1988) 248

Baggish, M.S., R Baltoyannis: New techniques for laser ablation of the endometrium in high-risk patients. Am. J. Obstet. Gynecol. 159 (1988) 287

Bailey, G., R.L. Strub, R.C. Klein: Dextran-induced anaphylaxis. J. Amer. Med. Ass. 200 (1961) 889

Bank, E.B.: Erfahrungen mit der Metroskopie, Zbl. Gynäkol. 82 (1960) 866

Barbaro, C.A., D.W. Fortune, A.S. Body, E. Henessy: Uterine lavage in the diagnostic of endometrial malignancy and its precursors. Acta cytol. 2 (1982) 135

Barbot, J., B. Parent, J.B. Dubuisson: Contact hysteroscopy: Another method of endoscopic examination of the uterine cavity. Am. J. Obstet. Gynecol. 136 (1980) 721

Bardt, J., L. Belkien, T. Vancaillie, C. Stening, H.P.G. Schneider: Ergebnisse diagnostischer Hysteroskopien in einem IVF/ET-Programm. Geburtsh. u. Frauenheilk. 44 (1984) 813

Berg, J.W., G.R. Durfee: The cytological presentation of endometrial carcinoma. Cancer 11 (1958) 158

Berle, P.: Fehlgeburt. In K.H. Wulf, H. Schmidt-Matthiesen: Klinik der Frauenheilkunde und Geburtshilfe. 3 (1985) 111

Beuttner, O.: Über Hysteroskopie. Zbl. Gynäkol. 22 (1898) 580

Bibbo, M., F.R. Reale, J. Reale, F. Azizi, P.H. Bartels, G.L. Wied, S.N. Hajj, A.L. Herbst: Assessment of three sampling technics to detect endometrial cancer and its precursors. Acta cytol. 23 (1979) 353

Bichler, K.-H., V. Ideler, P. Zöfel, R. Harzmann: Experimentelle Untersuchungen zur Hämolyse bei transurethralen Eingriffen. Urologe (A) 24 (1985) 229

Bitsch, M., K.J. Neis, N.K. Schöndorf, S. Bitsch: Vergleichende Studie von 4 Instrumenten zur intrauterinen Zellgewinnung nach der Bürstentechnik. Kurzfassung der Dreiländertagung für Klinische Zytologie. Hrsg. v. J.H. Holzner, K. Czerwenka. Robidruck, Wien 1984 (S. 57)

Bonte, J.: Diagnosis and treatment of precancerous endometrial lesions. In K.D. Schulz, R. King, K. Pollow, R. Taylor: Endometrial Cancer. Zuckschwerdt, München 1987 (S. 26)

Borten, M., C.P. Seibert, M.L. Taymor: Recurrent anaphylactic reaction to intraperitoneal dextran 75 used for prevention of postsurgical adhesions. Obstet. Gynecol. 61 (1983) 755

Boschann, H.W.: Cytomorphology of normal endometrium. Acta cytol. 2 (1958) 505

Boschann, H.W.: Cytometry on normal and abnormal endometrial cells. Acta cytol. 2 (1958) 520

Bozzini, P.: Der Lichtleiter oder Beschreibung einer einfachen Vorrichtung und ihrer Anwendung zur Erleuchtung innerer Höhlen und Zwischenräume des lebenden animalischen Körpers. Landes-Industrie-Comptoir, Weimar 1807

Braendle, W: Hysteroscopic evaluation of precancerous endometrial lesions. In H. Van der Pas, B. Van Herendael, D.A.F. Van Lith, L. Keith: Hysteroscopy. MTP Press, Boston 1983

Brandner, P., J. Gnirs, K.J. Neis, A. Hettenbach, W. Schmidt: Der Stellenwert der Vaginosonographie in der non-invasiven Beurteilung des Endometriums am postmenopausalen Uterus. Geburtsh. Frauenheilk. 51 (1991) 734-740

Brandner, P., K.J. Neis, G. Bastert: Vaginalsonographie am postmenopausalen Uterus: Die non-invasive Früherkennung von Neoplasien. Arch. Gynecol. Obstet. 245 (1989) 569

Brooks, P.G., S.P. Serden: Endometrial ablation in women with abnormal uterine bleeding aged fifty and over. J. Reprod. Med. 37 (1992) 682

Brooks, P.G., S.P Serden: Hysteroscopic findings after unsuccessful dilatation and curettage for abnormal uterine bleeding. Am. J. Obstet. Gynecol. 158 (1988) 1354

Brooks, P.G., F.D. Loffer, S.P. Serden: Resectoscopic removal of symptomatic intrauterine lesions. J. Reprod. Med. 34 (1989) 435

Brueschke, E.E., J.E. Fadel, K. Mayerhofer: Transcervical tubal occlusion with a steerable hysteroscope: implantation of devices into extirpated human uteri. Am. J. Obstet. Gynecol. 127 (1977) 118

Brun, G., R. Roussilhes, J. Saurel: Endometrectomie pour metrorrhagies: 45 cas. J. Gynecol. Obstet. Biol. Reprod. Paris 20 (1991) 532

Brundin, J.O.: P-block as a contraceptive method. In H. Van der Pas, B. Van Herendael, D.A.F. Van Lith, L. Keith: Hysteroscopy. MTP Press, Boston 1983

Brundin, J.O.: Experience with the P-block, an hidrogelic tubal blocking device. In A.M. Siegler, H.J. Lindemann: Hysteroscopy: Principles and Practice. Lippincott, Philadelphia 1984

Brundin, J.O.: Observations on the mode of action of an intratubal device, the P-block. Am. J. Obstet. Gynecol. 156 (1987) 997

Buchholz, F., G. Bonatz, K. Semm: Possibilities and limits of contact hysteroscopic assessment of the causes of postmenopausal bleeding. Zbl. Gynäkol. 10, 14 (1988) 884-889

Bumm, E.: Diskussion über die Endometritis. In R. Chrobak, I. Pfannestriel: Verhandlungen der Deutschen Gesellschaft für Gynäkologie. Breitkopf & Hartel, 1895 (p. 524)

Bumm, E.: Experimente und Erfahrungen mit der Hysteroskopie. In R. Chrobak, I. Pfannestriel: Verhandlungen der Deutschen Gesellschaft für Gynäkologie. Breitkopf & Hartel, 1895 (p. 524)

Burghardt, E.: Histologische Frühdiagnose des Zervixkrebses. Lehrbuch und Atlas. Thieme, Stuttgart 1972

Burkhart, S.S., C.R. Barmnett, S.J. Snyder: Transient postoperative blindness as a possible effect of glycine toxicity. Arthroscopy 6 (1990) 112

Burmucic, R., H.O. Mayer, R. Kömetter: Diagnosis and treatment of an occult intrauterine device. Wien med. Wschr. 137 (1987) 104

Burnett, J.E.: Hysteroscopy-controlled curettage for endometrial polyps. Obstet. Gynecol. 24 (1964) 621

Campo, R., J. Hucke: Die moderne diagnostische und operative Hysteroskopie. Workshopsyllabus des Leuven Institute for Fertility and Embryology, Leuven, Belgium und der Universitätsfrauenklinik Düsseldorf, Selbstverlag 1993

Campo, R.L., F. De Bruyne, J. Hucke: Neue diagnostische und therapeutische Verfahren in der Reproduktionsmedizin. Gynäkologe 23 (1990) 214

Caniels, B., W. Hammans, J. Landowski: Langzeitstudie zur endometrialen Zellgewinnung und zytologischen Beurteilbarkeit unter besonderer Berücksichtigung vom Prevical und Curity. Geburtsh. Frauenheilk. 45 (1985)

Carabias, J., V. Jr. Font-Sastre, F. Bonilla-Musoles, A. Pellicer: Atlas de histoscopia. Jims, Barcelona 1985

Carson, S.A., G.D. Hubert, E.D. Schriock, J.E. Buster: Hyperglycemia and hyponatremia during operative hysteroscopy with 5% dextrose in water distension. Fertil. Steril. 51 (1989) 341

Chervenak, F.A., R.S. Neuwirth: Hysteroscopic resection of the uterine septum. Am. J. Obstet. Gynecol 141 (1981) 351

Choban, M.J., S.B. Kalhan, R.J. Anderson, R. Collins: Pulmonary edema and coagulopathy following intrauterine instillation of 32 % dextran-70 (Hyskon). J. Clin. Anaesth. 3 (1991) 317

Choe, J.K., M.S. Baggish: Hysteroscopic treatment of septate uterus with Neodymium-YAG laser. Fertil. Steril. 57 (1992) 81

Cittadini, E., A. Perino, D. Gullo: Hysteroscopic endometrial patterns during replacement estrogen therapy. In A.M. Siegler, H.J. Lindemann: Hysteroscopy: Principles and Practice. Lippincott, Philadelphia 1984

Clocuh, Y.PA., C. Peters-Velte, F. Fischbach, P. Krieglsteiner: Ergebnisse zytologischer Untersuchungen von direkt entnommenem Zellmaterial aus dem Uteruscavum mit der Exploret-Fatol. Geburtsh. Frauenheilk. 42 (1982) 39

Cooper, J.M., R.M. Houck, H.S. Rigberg: The incidence of intrauterine abnormalities found at hysteroscopy in patients undergoing elective hysteroscopic sterilization. J. Reprod. Med. 28 (1983) 659

Cooper, J.M., R. Houck: Hysteroscopic tubal sterilization and formed-in-place silicone rubber plugs: cause significance and prevention of abnormal plugs. In A.M. Siegler, H.J. Lindemann: Hysteroscopy: Principles and Practice. Lippincott, Philadelphia 1984

Copperman, A.B., A.H DeCherney, D.L. Olive: A case of endometrial cancer following endometrial ablation for dysfunctional uterine bleeding. Obstet. Gynecol. 82 (1993) 640

Corson, S.L., F.R. Bather: CO_2 uterine distension for hysteroscopic septal incision. J. Reprod. Med. 31 (1986) 710

Craft, I.L.: Uterotubal ceramic plugs. In J.J. Sciarra, W. Droegemueller, J.J. Speidel: Advances in female sterilization techniques. Harper & Row, Hagerstorwn 1976 (p. 176)

Creasman, W.T., J. Lukeman: Role of the fallopian tube in dissemination of malignant cells in corpus cancer. Cancer 29 (1972) 456

Creasman, W.T., J.C. Wedd: Screening technique in endometrial cancer. Cancer 38 (1976) 436

Creevy, C.D.: Hemolytic reactions during transurethral prostatic resections. J. Urol. 58 (1947) 125

Crippa, L.: Letter to Editor. Cervix 4 (1986) 101

Christopherson, W.M., R.C. Alherhasky, P.J. Connelly: Carcinoma of the endometrium I, a clinicopathologic study of clear cell carcinoma and secretory carcinoma. Cancer 49 (1982) 1511

Christopherson, W.M., R.C. Alherhasky, P.J. Connelly: Carcinoma of the endometrium II, papillary adenocarcinoma. Am. J. Clin. Pathol. 77 (1982) 534

Cronje H.S., C.J. Deale: Staging of endometrial cancer by hysteroscopy. S. Afr. Med. J. 73, 12 (1988) 716-717

Crozier, T.A., A. Luger, M. Dravec, M. Sydow, J. Radke, W. Rath, W. Kuhn, D. Kettler: Gasembolie mit Kreislaufstillstand bei Hysteroskopien: Fallberichte von drei Patientinnen. Anästhesiol. Intensivmed. Notfallmed. Schmerzther. 26 (1991) 412

Dachs, G.: Praktikabilität der Jetwash-Technik. Inauguraldiss., Hamburg 1980

Dallenbach-Hellweg, G., H. Schmidt-Matthiesen: Hyperplasien, Präcancerosen und Carcinome des Endometriums. Gynäkol. Geburtsh. 4 (1983) 13

Dallenbach-Hellweg. G., H. Poulsen: Atlas der Histopathologie des Endometriums. Springer, Berlin 1984

Daly, D.C., C.A. Walters, C.E. Soto-Albors, H.D. Riddick: Hysteroscopic metroplasty: surgical technique and obstetric outcome. Fertil. Steril. 39 (1983) 623

Daly, D.C., D. Maier, C. Soto-Albors: Hysteroscopic metroplasty: six years' experience. Obstet. Gynecol. 73 (1989) 201

Daniell, J., R. Tosh, S. Meisels: Photodynamic ablation of the endometrium with the Nd: YAG Laser hysteroscopically as a treatment for menorrhagia. Colpos Gynecol. Laser Surg. 2 (1986) 43

Darabi, K.F., R.M. Richard: Collaborative Study on Hysteroscopic Sterilization Procedures. Preliminary Report. Obstet. Gynecol. 49 (1977) 48

David, A., L. Mettler, K. Semm: The cervical polyp: A new diagnostic and therapeutic approach with CO_2 hysteroscopy. Am. J. Obstet. Gynecol. 130 (1978) 662

David, C. L'endoscopie uterine (hysteroscopie). Thèse, Paris, G. Jaques, Publisher. No. 112

Davies, J.A.: Hysteroscopic endometrial ablation with the neodymium-YAG laser. Brit. J. Obstet. Gynaecol. 96 (1989) 928

Davis, R.H., R.A. Erb, G.A., Kyriazis: Fallopian tube occlusion in rabbits with silicone rubber. J. Reprod. Med. 14 (1975) 56

Davis, R.H., H.A. Platt, D.K. Moonka: Chronic occlusion of the monkey fallopian tube with silicone polymer. Obstet. Gynecol. 53 (1979) 527

Deaton J.L., D. Maier, J. Jr. Andreoli: Spontaneous uterine rupture during pregnancy after treatment of Asherman's syndrome. Am. J. Obstet. Gynecol. 160 (1989) 1053

DeCherney, A.H.: Hysteroscopic management of Müllerian fusion defects. In A.M. Siegler, H.J. Lindemann: Hysteroscopy: Principles and Practice. Lippincott, Philadelphia 1984, p. 204

DeCherney, A.H., I. Cholst, F. Naftolin: The management of intractable uterine bleeding utilizing the cystoscopic resectope. In A.M. Siegler, H.J. Lindemann: Hysteroscopy: Principles and Practice. Lippincott, Philadelphia 1984: 140

DeCherney, A.H., M.P Diamond, G. Lavy, M.L. Polan: Endometrial ablation for intractable uterine bleeding: hysteroscopic resection. Obstet. Gynecol. 70 (1987) 668

DeCherney, A.H., M.L. Polan: Hysteroscopic management of intrauterine lesions and intractable uterine bleeding. Obstet. Gynecol. 61 (1983) 392

De Mayer, J.F.D.E.: Transcervikal hysteroscopic sterilization. In H. Van der Pas, B. van Herendael, D.A.F. Van Lith, L. Keith: Hysteroscopy. MTP Press, Boston 1983

De Mayer, J.F.D.E.: Hysteroscopic sterilization with silicone rubber: a review of 3 and a half years experience. In A.M. Siegler, H.J. Lindemann: Hysteroscopy: Principles and Practice, Lippincott, Philadelphia 1984

Dequesne, J.: Hysteroscopic therapy of uterine bleeding with the Nd:YAG-laser. Laser Med. Sci. 2 (1987) 73

Deligdisch, L., C.J. Cohen: Histologic correlates and virulence implications of endometrical carcinoma associated with adenomatous hyperplasia. Cancer 56 (1985) 1452

Desormeaux, A.J.: De l'endoscope et de ses applications au diagnostic et au traitement des affections de l'urètre et de la vessie. Bailliire, Paris 1865

Deutschmann, C., R.P. Lueken, H.J. Lindemann: Hysteroscopic findings in postmenopausal bleeding. In A.M. Siegler, H.J. Lindemann: Hysteroscopy: Principles and Practice. Lippincott, Philadelphia 1983

Deutschmann, C., Lueken R.P.: Hysteroscopic findings in postmenopausal bleeding. In A.M. Siegler, H.J. Lindemann: Hysteroscopy: Principles and Practice. Lippincott, Philadelphia 1984 (p. 132)

Devi, P.K., A.N. Kupta: Hysteroscopic removal of intrauterine contraceptive devices with missing threads. Indian J. Med. 65 (1977) 5

Dexeus, S., R. Labastida, A. Arias: Hysteroscopy in abnormal uterine bleeding. In A.M. Siegler, H.J. Lindemann: Hysteroscopy: Principles and Practice. Lippincott, Philadelphia 1984 (p. 123)

Dexeus, S., R. Labastida, L. Marques: Hysteroscopy in daily gynecologic practice. Acta Europ. Fertil. 17 (1986) 6

Dicker, R., J. Greenspan, L. Straus: Complications of abdominal and vaginal hysterectomy among women of reproductive age in the United States. Am. J. Obstet. Gynecol. 144 (1982) 841

DiSaia, P.J., P.C. Morrow, W.T. Creasman, R. Kurman: GOG Protocol Nr. 33. In Gynecologic oncology group. Statistical Report (1982)

Dolff, M.: Carbon dioxide hysteroscopy before tubal microsurgery. In A.M. Siegler, H.J. Lindemann: Hysteroscopy: Principles and Practice. Lippincott, Philadelphia 1984

Donnez, J., M. Nisolle: Hysteroscopic surgery. Curr. Opin. Obstet. Gynecol. 4 (1992) 439

Donnez, J., S. Gillerot, D. Bourgonjon, F. Clercks, M. Nisolle: Neodymium:YAG laser hysteroscopy in large submucous fibroids. Fertil. Steril. 43 (1990): 999

Donnez, J., B. Schrurs, S. Gillerot, J. Sandow, F. Clerckx: Treatment of uterine fibroids with implants of gonadotropin-releasing hormone agonist: assessment by hysterography. Fertil. Steril. 51 (1989) 947

Droegemueller, W., B.E. Greet, E. Makowski: Cryosurgery in patients with dysfunctional uterine bleeding. Obstet. Gynecol. 38 (1971) 256

Droegemueller, W., B.E. Greet, J.R. David: Cryocoagulation of the endometrium at the uterine cornua. Am. J. Obstet. Gynecol. 131 (1978) 1

Druhl, S., H.J. Lindemann, J. Mohr: Erste Erfahrungen mit einer neuen Thermosonde für die transuterine Tubensterilisation. Arch. Gynäkol. 219 (1975) 39

Druhl, S., H.J. Lindemann: Sterilität der Frau: organische Ursachen. Diagnostik 9 (1976) 50

ECRI: Fatal gas embolism associated with intrauterine laser surgery. Health Devices 18 (1989): 325

Edström, K., I. Fernström: The diagnostic possibilities of a modified hysteroscopic technique. Acta Obstet. Gynecol. Scand. 49 (1970) 327

Englund, S., A. Ingelmann-Sundberg, B. Westin: Hysteroscopy in diagnosis and treatment of uterine bleeding. Gynecologia 143 (1957) 217

Erb, R.A.: Hysteroscopic sterilization with formed-in-place silicone rubber plugs. Basic process and instruments. In A.M. Siegler, H.J. Lindemann: Hysteroscopy: Principles and Practice. Lippincott, Philadelphia 1984

Esposito, A., G. Accinelli: Praktische Anwendung der Hysteroskopie in der Gynäkologie. Zbl. Gynäkol. 88 (1966) 1676

Fayez, J.A.: Comparison between abdominal and hysteroscopic metroplasty. Obstet. Gynecol. 68 (1986) 399

Fayez, J.A., G. Mutie, P.J. Schneider: The diagnostic value of hysterosalpingography and hysteroscopy in infertility investigation. Am. J. Obstet. Gynecol. 156 (1987) 558

FDA Drug Bulletin. Users reminded about adverse reactions to dextran. 13 (1983) 23

Fedele, L., E. Ferrazzi, M. Dorta, P. Vercellini, G.B. Candiani: Ultrasonography in the differential diagnosis of "double" uteri. Fertil. Steril. 50 (1988) 361

Fedele, L., P. Vercellini, T. Viezoli, O. Ricciardiello, D. Zamberletti: Intrauterine adhesions: current diagnostic and therapeutic trends. Acta Eur. Fertil. 17 (1986) 31

Feichter, G.E., P.F. Tauber: Zytologische Endometrium-Diagnostik mit Prevical. Fortschr. Med. 24 (1981) 94

Feichter, G.E., P.F Tauber, J. Landowski: Clinical experience with a new endometrial cell sampling kit (Isaacs cell sampler). Acta cytol. 26 (1982) 141

Filshie, G.M., K.H. Nicolaides: Cervical dilatation with lamicel prior to hysteroscopy. In H. Van der Pas, B. Van Herendael, D. Van Lith, C. Keith: Hysteroscopy. MTP Press, Boston 1983 (p. 33)

Fitzpatrick, J.M., P.P. Kasidas, G.A. Rose: Hyperoxaluria following glycine irrigation for transurethral prostatectomy. Br. J. Urol. 53 (1981) 250

Foley D.V., T. Masukawa: Endometrial monitoring of high-risk women. Cancer 48 (1981) 511

Freund, A.: Ein neues, mit Curette verbundenes Uterusendoskop. Geburtshilfe Gynäkol. 91 (1927) 663

Frydman, R., C. Gerodolle, J.E. Hamou: Interest of microhysteroscopy before in vitro fertilization. Acta Europ. Fertil. 17 (1986) 453

Gallinat, A.: Endometriumablation unter Verwendung des Neodym-Yag Lasers bei der CO_2 Hysteroskopie. In: Endoscopic surgery in gynecology, Lueken, R.P., A. Gallinat (Hrsg.), Dememter Verlag Gräfelfing (1992) 117

Gallinat, A.: Hysteroskopische Behandlung submuköser Myome durch den Einsatz des Nd:Yag-Laser und moderner Elektrotechnik. In: Endoscopic surgery in gynecology, Lueken, R.P., A. Gallinat (Hrsg.), Dememter Verlag Gräfelfing (1992) 76

Gallinat, A.: The effect of carbon dioxide during hysteroscopy. In H. Van der Pas, B. Van Herendael, D.A.F. Van Lith, L. Keith: Hysteroscopy. MTP Press, Boston 1983

Gallinat, A.: Hysteroscopy as a diagnostic and therapeutic procedure in sterility. In A.M. Siegler, H.J. Lindemann: Hysteroscopy: Principles and Practice. Lippincott, Philadelphia 1984 (p. 180)

Gallinat, A.: Hysteroscopy in early pregnancy. In A.M. Siegler, H.J. Lindemann: Hysteroscopy: Principles and Practice. Lippincott, Philadelphia 1984

Gallinat, A., R.P. Luken, H.J. Lindemann: Komplikationen mit Intrauterinpessaren. Sexualmedizin 7 (1978) 215

Gamerre, M., H. Serment: Hysteroscopy vs. hysterosgraphy. In H. Van der Pas, B. Van Herendael, D.A.F. Van Lith, L. Keith: Hysteroscopy. MTP Press, Boston 1983

Garmanova, N.V., L.I. Dekster, A.F. Urmancheeva et al.: Endoscopic study methods in the diagnosis of the initial forms of cervical cancer in pregnant women. Vop. Onkol. 27 (1981) 72

Gaus, C.J.: Hysteroskopie. Arch. Gynäkol. 133 (1928) 18

Gaus, C.J.: Hysteroskopie. Verh.phys.-med. Ges. Würzb. 52 (1927) 99

Gentile, G.P., A.M. Siegler: Inadvertent intestinal biopsy during laparoscopy and hysteroscopy. A report of two cases. Fertil. Steril. 36 (1981) 402

Getzen, J.H., W. Speiggle: Anaphylactic reaction to dextran. Arch. intern. Med. 112 (1963) 168

Gimpelson, R.J.: Panoramic hysteroscopy with directed biopsis vs. dilatation and curettage for accurate Diagnosis. J. Reprod. Med. 29 (1984) 575

Gimpelson, R.J., H.O. Rappold: A comparative study between panoramic hysteroscopy with directed biopsis and dilatation and curettage. A review of 276 cases. Am. J. Obstet. Gynecol. 158 (1988) 489

Golan, A., R. Langer, I. Bukovsky, E. Caspi: Congenital anomalies of the müllerian system. Fertil. Steril. 51, 5 (1989) 747

Goldrath, M.H., T.A. Fuller, S. Segal: Laser photovaporization of endometrium for the treatment of menorrhagia. Am. J. Obstet. Gynecol. 140 (1981) 14

Goldrath, M.H., A.I. Sherman: Office hysteroscopy and suction curettage: can we eliminate hospital diagnostic dilatation and curettage? Am. J. Obstet. Gynecol. 152 (1984) 220

Gravlee, L.C.: Jet-irrigation method for the cytologic diagnosis of endometrial adenocarcinoma. Its principle and accuracy. Obstet. Gynecol. 34 (1969) 168

Greene, L.F.: Komplikationen bei der transurethralen Resektion des Prostataadenoms. Extracta Urologica 5 (1981) 13

Gresenhues, T., R. Hackenberg, U. Deichert, G. Sturm, K.D. Schulz: Treatment of uterine fibroids with the GnRH-analogue Goserelin. Gynecol. Endocrinol. 4 (1990) 41

Grosspietzsch, R., W. Husstedt, F. Oberheuser: Uterus-Perforation durch Intrauterinpessar. Pädiat. Prax. 19 (1978) 513

Gupta, I., P.K. Devi, A.N. Gupta: Hysteroscopic removal of intrauterine devices with missing threads. Indian. J. Med. Res. 65 (1977) 661

Hackenberg, R., T. Gresenhues, U. Deichert, V. Duda, G. Sturm, K.D. Schulz: Präoperative Reduktion von Uterusmyomen durch das GnRH-Analogon Goserelin (Zoladex). Geburtsh. Frauenheilk. 50 (1990) 136

Hahn, R.G., J.C. Ekengren: Patterns of irrigating fluid absorption during transurethral resection of the prostate as indicated by ethanol. J. Urol. 149 (1993) 502

Hahn, R.G.: Serum amino acid patterns and toxicity symptoms following the absorption of irrigant containing gylcine in transurethral prostatic surgery. Acta Anaesthesiol. Scand. 32 (1988) 493

Hald, F., S.E. Kristoffersen, E. Gregersen: Prostaglandin vaginal suppositories in non pregnant women requiring cervical dilatation prior to hysteroscopy. Acta Obstet. Gynecol. Scand. 67 (1988) 219

Hallez, J.P., A. Netter, R. Cartier: Methodical intrauterine resection. Am. J. Obstet. Gynecol. 131 (1978) 91

Hamou, J.E.: Microhysteroscopy. Acta Endosc. 10 (1980) 415

Hamou, J.E.: Hystéroscopie et microhystéroscopie avec un instrument nouveau: Le microhystéroscope. Endosc. Gynécol. 2 (1980) 131

Hamou, J.E.: Microhysteroscopy. A new procedure and it's original applications in gynecology. J. Reprod. Med. 26 (1981) 375

Hamou, J.E., J. Salat-Baroux, F. Coupez: La microhystéroscopie dans la détection du carcinome intraépithelial. In de Bichat: Expansion Scientifique Française. Serment, Paris 1981 (p. 179)

Hamou, J.: Microhystéroscopie: Mises à Jour Collège Français. Vigot Press, Paris 1981

Hamou, J.E., P.J. Tayler: Panoramic, contact, and microcolpohysteroscopy in gynecology. Practice. In Current Problems in Obstet. Gynecol. Year Book Medical Publishes, Chicago 6 (1982) 2

Hamou, J.E., J. Salat-Baroux, A.M. Siegler: Diagnosis and management of intrauterine adhesions by microhysteroscopy. Fertil. Steril. 39 (1983) 321

Hamou, J.E.: In-vivo-Zytologie-Histologie mit der Kolpo-Mikro-Hysteroskopie. Vortrag 45. Tagung der Deutschen Gesellschaft für Gynäkologie und Geburtshilfe, Frankfurt 1984

Hamou, J.E., J. Salat-Baroux: Advanced hysteroscopy and microhysteroscopy in 1,000 patients. In A.M. Siegler, H.J. Lindemann: Hysteroscopy: Principles and Practice. Lippincott, Philadelphia 1984

Hartmann, M.: Erfahrungen mit Purisole SM bei transurethralen Elektroresektionen. Urologe 19 (1979) 232

Harzmann, R., K. van Deyk: Nichtinvasive Erfassung des TUR-Syndroms bei transurethralen Resektionen. Akt. Nephrol. 3 (1982) 410

Haselbach, U., K.J. Neis, S. Riehm, G. Bastert: Immuncytochemische Darstellung des Ostrogenrezeptors und Progesteronrezeptors am Endometrium unter physiologischen Bedingungen. Arch. Gynecol. Obstet. 245 (1989) 586

Haselgorst, G.: Unsere Erfahrungen mit der Hysteroskopie. Zbl. Gynäkol. 59 (1935) 2442

Healy, D.L.: The use of LHRH agonists in treating uterine fibroids. Gynecol. Endocrinol., 2 Suppl. 1 (1988) 26

Healy, D.L., H.M. Fraser, S.L. Lawson: Shrinkage of a uterine fibroid after subcutaneous infusion of a LH-RH agonist. Br. Med. J. 209 (1984) 267

Hendrickson, M.R., R.L. Kempson: Surgical pathology of the uterine corpus. Major problems in pathology, Vol. 12. Saunders, Philadelphia 1980

Hepp, H.: Die gynäkologische Endoskopie. 11. Hysteroskopie und Amnioskopie. Dtsch. Ärztebl. 71 (1974) 2525

Hepp, H., H. Roll: Die Hysteroskopie. Gynäkologe 7 (1974) 166

Hepp, H., G. Hoffmann, R. Kreienberg: Möglichkeiten und Grenzen der Hysteroskopie in der Diagnostik des Corpuscarcinoms. Fortschr. Med. 95 (1977) 2113

Hepp, H.: Zum Problem des "verlorenen" Intrauterinpessars. Geburtsh. u. Frauenheilk. 37 (1977) 653

Hepp, H.: Diagnostics in hysteroscopy. Endoscopy 10 (1978) 232

Hepp, H., G. Hoffmann, R. Kreienberg, P. Brockerhof: Indikationen zur Hysteroskopie bei der Diagnostik des Corpuscarcinoms. Gynäkol. Prax. 2 (1978) 81

Hepp, H.: Vermeidung von Komplikationen bei der gynäkologischen Laparoskopie und Hysteroskopie. In Beck: Intraund postoperative Komplikationen in der Gynäkologie. Thieme, Stuttgart 1979

Hepp, H., K.J. Neis: Problematik der operativen Therapie des Corpuscarcinoms. 22. Fortbildungstagung in den Dr.-Horst-Schmidt-Kliniken, Klinikum der Landeshauptstadt Wiesbaden Frauenklinik. Berle, Wiesbaden 1983

Hillemanns, H.: Entstehung und Wachstum des Zervixkarzinoms. Fortsch. Geburtsh. Gynäkol., Bd. 18, Karger, Basel 1964

Hinselmanns, H.: Die Kolposkopie. Girardet, Wuppertal-Elberfeld 1954

Hoekstra, P.T., R. Kahnoski, M.A. McCamish, W. Bergen, D.R. Heetderks: Transurethral prostatic resection syndrome—a new perspective: encephalopathy with associated hyperammonemia. J. Urol. 130 (1983): 704

Holzgreve, W., R Miny, C. Stening, T.H. Vancaille, F.K. Beller: Experience with different techniques of chorionic villi sampling for first trimester diagnosis. Acta Europ. Fertil. 17 (1986) 485

Hucke, J., F. DeBruyne, R.L. Campo, A.A. Freikha: Hysteroscopic treatment of congenital uterine malformations causing hemihematometra: a report of three cases. Fertil. Steril. 58 (1992) 823

Hucke, J., R.L. Campo, F. DeBruyne: Schwangerschaft nach kombiniert mikrochirurgischem und operativ-hysteroskopischem Vorgehen bei einer Patientin mit Uterus septus und Vagina septa. Geburtsh. Frauenheilk 51 (1991) 486

Hucke, J., R.L. Campo, F. DeBruyne, A. Abou Freikha: Die hysteroskopische Resektion submuköser Myome. Geburtsh. Frauenheilk. 52 (1992) 214

Hull, C.H., H.H. Nie: SPSS-Update. New procedures and facilities for release 7 and 9. McGraw-Hill, New York 1979

Iglesias, J.J., U.K. Stams: Hämolyse ist nicht Ursache des TUR-Syndroms. Die Verwendung nicht hämolysierender Spüllösungen kann es nicht verhindern. Urologe 14 (1975) 292

Indman, P.D., W.W. Brown: Uterine surface temperature changes caused by electrosurgical endometrial coagulation. J. Reprod. Med. 37 (1992) 667

Indman, P.D., Hysteroscopic treatment of menorrhagia associated with uterine leiomyomas. Obstet. Gynecol. 81 (1993) 716

Isaacs, J.H., F.H. Ross: Cytologic evaluation of the endometrium in woman with postmenopausal bleeding. Am. J. Obstet. Gynecol. 131 (1978)

Itzkowic, D., M. Beale: Uterine perforation associated with endometrial ablation. Aust. N.Z.J. Obstet. Gynecol. 32 (1992) 359

Jedeikin, R., D. Olsfanger, I. Kessler: Disseminated intravascular coagulopathy and adult respiratory distress syndrome: Life-threatening complications of hysteroscopy. Am. J. Obstet. Gynecol. 162 (1990) 44

Jiminez-Ayala, M., E. Vilaplana, C.B. De Bengoa, M. Zomeno. E. Moreno, M. Granados: Endometrial and endocervical brushing techniques with a Medhosa cannula. Acta cytol. 19 (1975) 557

Joelsson, I.S., R.U. Levine, G. Moberger: Hysteroscopy as an adjunct in determining the extent of carcinoma of the endometrium. Am. J. Obstet. Gynecol. 111 (1971) 696

Joelsson, I.S.: Hysteroscopy for delineating the intrauterine extent of endometrial carcinoma. In A.M. Siegler, H.J. Lindemann: Hysteroscopy: Principles and Practice. Lippincott, Philadelphia 1984 (p. 154)

Johnson, J.E.: Hysterography and diagnostic curettage in carcinoma of the uterine body. Acta Radiol. 326 (1973) 1

Jordan, M., G. Bader, Nemazie, B. Karacz: Comparative accuracy of preoperativ cytologic and histologic diagnosis in endometrial lesions. Obstet. Gynecol. 7 (1956) 611

Juricic, D., Z. Al-Naieb, C.F. Hoffmann, U. Engelmann: Spüllösungen in der Endoskopie. Uroscop 1/89

Kern, G., J.P. Nolens: Langzeitbeobachtungen von dysplastischem und gesteigert atypischem Epithel. Arch. Gynäk. 207 (1969) 342

Khalifa, E., J.P. Toner, H.W. Jones Jr.: The role of abdominal metroplasty in the era of operative hysteroscopy. Surg. Gynecol. Obstet. 176 (1993) 208

Knudtson, M.L., P.J. Tayler: Überempfindlichkeitsreaktion auf Dextran 70 (Hyskon) während einer Hysteroskopie. Geburtsh. u. Frauenheilk. 36 (1976) 263

Kofler, E., E. Reinhold, R. Ulm, P. Wagenbichler: Möglichkeiten und Grenzen der zytologischen Diagnostik des Carcinom adenomatosum uteri. Fortschr. Med. 88 (1970) 733

Kontopoulos, V.: Hysteroscopic lysis of intrauterine adhesions: a report of 61 cases. Acta Europ. Fertil. 17 (1986) 473

Koss, L.G.: Cytologic diagnosis of carcinoma of the uterine cervix. In L.A. Gray: Dysplasia, carcinoma in situ and micro-invasive carcinoma of the cervix uteri. Thomas, Springfield (1964) p. 190

Koss, L.G., G.R. Durfee: Cytologic diagnosis of endometrial carcinoma. Results of ten years experience. Acta cytol. 6 (1962) 519

Koss, L.G., K. Schreiber, S.G. Oberlander, M. Moukhtar, H.S. Lenine, H.F. Moussouris: Srceening of asymptomatic women for endometrial cancer. Obstet. Gynecol. 57 (1981) 681

Koss, L.G., K. Schreiber, S.G. Oberlander, H.F. Moussouris, M. Lesser: Detection of endometrial carcinoma and hyperplasia in asymptomic women. Obstet. Gynecol. 64 (1984) 1

Kottmeier, H.L.: Annual report on the results of treatment in gynecological cancer. Stockholm 19 (1985)

Kula, K., A. Flariewicz-Kula: Physiology of sperm migration and its importance in the methodology of artificial insemination with special reference to hysteroscopy. In H. Van der Pas, B. Van Herendael, D.A.F. Van Lith, L. Keith: Hysteroscopy. MTP Press, Boston 1983 (p. 211)

Kullander, S., B. Sandahl: Fetal chromosome analysis after transcervical placental biopsies during early pregnancy. Acta Obstet. Gynecol. Scand. 52 (1973) 355

Kurman, R.J.: Blaustein's Pathology of the Female Genital Tract, 3. Springer, Berlin 1987

Kurman, R.J., H.J. Norris: Endometrial carcinoma. In R.J. Kurmann Blaustein's Pathology of the Female Genital Tract, 3rd ed., Springer, Berlin 1987 (p. 338)

Labastida, R., S. Dexeus, A. Arias: Hysteroscopy in abnormal uterine bleeding. In H. Van der Pas, B. Van Herendael, D. Van Lith, C. Keith: Hysteroscopy. MTP Press, Boston 1983 (115)

Labastida, R., S. Dexeui, A. Arias: infertility and hysteroscopy. In A.M. Siegler, H.J. Lindemann: Hysteroscopy: Principles and Practice. Lippincott, Philadelphia, 1984 (p. 175)

Lange, H.J.: Statische und epidemiologische Aspekte der Früherkennung von Krankheiten. Vortrag anläßl. d. 7. Dreiländertagung für klin. Zytologie. Salzburg DÄV wissensch. Reihe 13 (1977)

La Sala, G.B., F. Sacchetti, L. Dessanti: Ambulatory diagnostic hysteroscopy: our experience with Hamou's microhysteroscopy in 676 patients. Am. J. Obstet. Gynecol. 5 (1984) 300

La Sala, G.B., F. Sacchetti, L. Dessanti: Isteroscopia diagnostica ambulatoriale: nostra esperienza con il microisterocopio di Hamou in 676 pazienti. Amer. Ost. Gin. Med. Perin. CV (1984) 300

La Sala, G.B., L. Dessanti, F. Sacchetti: Hysteroscopy and female sterility: analysis of the results from 213 patients. Acta Europ. Fertil. 16 (1985) 47

La Sala, G.B., F Sacchetti, E Degl'incertitocci, L. Dessanti, M.G. Torrelli: Complementary use of hysterosalpingography, hysteroscopy and laparoscopy in 100 infertile patients: results and comparison of their diagnostic accuracy. Acta Europ. Fertil. 18 (1987) 369

Leake, J.F., A.A. Murphy, H.A. Zacur: Noncardiogenic pulmonary edema: a complication of operative hysteroscopy. Fertil. Steril. 48 (1987) 497

Levine, R.U., G. Moberger: The extent of carcinoma of the endometrium. Am. J. Obstet. Gynecol. 111 (1971) 696

Levine,R.U., R.S. Neuwirth: Evaluation of a method of hysteroscopy with the use of 30 % dextran. Am. J. Obstet. Gynecol. 113 (1972) 696

Levine, R.U., R.S. Neuwirth: Simultaneous laparoscopy and hysteroscopy for intrauterine adhesions. Obstet. Gynecol. 42 (1973) 441

Lewis, G.C., B. Bundy: Surgery for endometrial cancer. Cancer 48 (1981) 568

Lindemann, H.J.: Eine neue Untersuchungsmethode für die Hysteroskopie. Endoscopy 4 (1971) 194

Lindemann, H.J.: Hysteroscopy for the diagnosis of intrauterine causes of sterility. Fertility and Sterility. New York 1971

Lindemann, H.J.: The use of CO_2 in the uterine cavity for hysteroscopy. Int. J. Fertil. 17 (1972) 221

Lindemann, H.J.: Hysteroskopie v suvise s planovanium rodicostva. Cs. Gynecol. 37 (1972) 7

Lindemann, H.J.: Eine neue Methode für die Hysteroskopie. Fortschr. Endosc. 4 (1973) 185

Lindemann, H.J.: Die Hysteroskopie. Arch. Gynäkol. 214 (1973) 241

Lindemann, H.J.: Uteroscopie. Med. Hyg. 1082 (1973) 1927

Lindemann, H.J.: Pneumometra für die Hysteroskopie. Geburtsh. Frauenheilk. 33 (1973) 18

Lindemann, H.J.: Transuterine Tubensterilisation per Hysteroskop. Geburtsh. Frauenheilk. 33 (1973) 709

Lindemann, H.J.: Historical aspects of hysteroscopy. Fertil. Steril. 24 (1973) 230

Lindemann, H.J.: Fortschritte, Risiken und Grenzen der Endoskopie in der Gynäkologie. Fortschr. Endosc. 5 (1974) 147

Lindemann, H.J.: Transuterine tubal sterilization by CO_2 hysteroscopy. In J.J. Sciarra, J.C. Beutler, J.J. Speidel: Hysteroscopic Sterilization. Intercont Med. Book, New York 1974 (p. 61)

Lindemann, H.J., J. Mohr: Ergebnisse von 274 transuterinen Tubensterilisationen per Hysteroskop. Geburtsh. Frauenheilk. 34 (1974) 775

Lindemann, H.J., J. Mohr: Die Hysteroskopie als Untersuchungsmethode Infertilität der Frau. Fortschr. Steril. 3 (1974) 102

Lindemann, H.J.: Die Wertigkeit der gynäkologischen Endoskopie gegenüber der Histologie und Zytologie. Fortschr. Endosc. 6 (1975) 63

Lindemann, H.J.: Komplikationen bei der CO_2-Hysteroskopie. Arch. Gynäcol. 219 (1975) 257

Lindemann, H.J.: Ergebnisse nach 230 transuterinen Tubensterilisationen per Hysteroskop. Fortschr. Endosc. 6 (1975) 153

Lindemann, H.J., A.M. Siegler, J. Mohr: The Hysteroflator 1000S. J. Reprod. Med. 16 (1976) 145

Lindemann, H.J., J. Mohr, A. Gallinat, M. Buros: Einfluß von CO_2-Gas während der Hysteroskopie. Geburtsh. Frauenheilk. 36 (1976) 153

Lindemann, H.J., A. Gallinat: Physikalische und physiologische Grundlagen der CO_2-Hysteroskopie. Geburtsh. Frauenheilk. 36 (1976) 729

Lindemann, H.J., J. Mohr: CO_2hysteroscopy: diagnosis and treatment. Am. J. Obstet Gynecol. 124 (1976) 124

Lindemann, H.J., S. Druhl: Diagnostik organischer Sterilitätsursachen der Frau. Diagnostik 9 (1976) 50

Lindemann, H.J.: Hysteroskopie. Gynäkol. Prax. 1 (1977) 455

Lindemann, H.J., R.P Lueken: Diagnosis and treatment of lost IUD's using CO_2-hysteroscopy. Endoscopy 9 (1977) 119

Lindemann, H.J., J. Mohr: CO_2-Hysteroskopie, eine Methode zur Entfernung okkulter Intrauterinpessare. Arch. Gynäkol. 224 (1977) 31

Lindemann, H.J., R.P. Lueken: Local and systematic administration of sulprostone for cervical dilatation in non-pregnant patients. In International Sulprostone Symposium in Vienna. Schering, Berlin 1978 (p. 65)

Lindemann, H.J.: Hysteroscopy-today and tomorrow. Endoscopy 10 (1978) 234

Lindemann, H.J., R.P. Lueken, A. Gallinat: Prenatale Diagnostik einer Doppelspaltbildung. Geburtsh. Frauenheilk. 38 (1978) 474

Lindemann, H.J.: Therapeutic possibilities with hysteroscopy. Endoscopy 10 (1978) 232

Lindemann, H.J.: CO₂-hysteroscopy today. Endoscopy 11 (1979) 94

Lindemann, H.J., A. Gallinat, R.P. Lueken: Metromat—a new instrument for producing pneumometra. J. Reprod. Med. 23 (1979)

Lindemann, H.J., A. Gallinat, R.P. Lueken, J. Mohr: Atlas der Hysteroskopie. Fischer, Stuttgart 1980

Lindemann, H.J., C.W. Popp, R.P. Lueken: Hysterosonographie. Diagn. u. Intensivmed. 4 (1982) 69

Lindemann, H.J.: The choice of distension medium in hysteroscopy. In H. Van der Pas, B. Van Herendael, D.A.F. Van Lith, L. Keith: Hysteroscopy. MTP Press, Boston 1983 (p. 11)

Lindemann, H.J., C.W. Popp, R.P. Lueken, W. Müller-Holve: Gynäkologische Endosonographie: Erste Erfahrungen. Ultraschall 4 (1983) 92

Lindemann, H.J.: Die Hysteroskopie in der Sterilitätsdiagnostik. Sterilität und Fertilität 1 (1985) 17

Lindemann, H.J.: Hysteroscopy for the transcervical resection of the septum uteri. Arch. Gynecol. 237 (1985) 196

Lindemann, H.J.: Die Endoskopie als Diagnostik und Therapie bei der kinderlosen Frau. Arch. Gynecol. 22 (1986) 9

Lindemann, H.J.: Safety commitee. The Hysteroscope, Newsletter of the European Society of Hysteroscopy 3 (1989) 3

Liukko, P., M. Grönroos, R. Punnonen, P. Kilkku: Methods for evaluating the intrauterine location of carcinoma. Acta Obstet. Gynecol. Scand. 58 (1979) 275

Loch, E.G., K. Frank, P. Linhart: Klinische Bedeutung der routinemäßigen sonographischen Untersuchungen in der Frauenheilkunde. Ultraschall 5 (1984) 1993

Loffer, F.D., P.S. Loffer: Will be the hysteroscopic silicone tubal plugs become a widely accepted technique? In A.M. Siegler, H.J. Lindemann: Hysteroscopy: Principles and Practice. Lippincott, Philadelphia, 1984

Loffer, F.D.: Hysteroscopic management of menorrhagia. Acta Europ. Fertil. 17 (1986) 463

Loffer, F.D.: Hysteroscopic endometrial ablation with the Nd:YAG laser using a nontouch technique. Obstet. Gynecol. 69 (1987) 679

Loffer, F.D.: Hysteroscopy with selective endometrial sampling compared with D&C for abnormal uterine bleeding: the value of a negative hysteroscopic view. Obstet. Gynecol. 73 (1989) 16

Loffer, F.D.: Complications form uterine distension during hysteroscopy. In: Complications of laparoscopy and hysteroscopy, Corfman, R.S., M.P. Diamond, A. DeCherney (eds), Blackwell Scientific Publications, Oxford (1993) 177

Loffer, F.D.: Fluid cooling of artificial saphire tips of laser. Am J. Obstet. Gynecol. 163 (1990) 681

Loft, A., T.F. Anderson, H. Bronnum-Hansen, C. Roepstorff, M. Madsen: Early postoperative mortality following hysterectomy. A Danish population study, 1977-1981. Br. J. Obstet, Gynaecol. 98 (1991) 147

Lohe, K.J., J. Baltzer: Weibliche Genitalorgane Teil I. In P. Hermanek: Kompendium der klinischen Tumorpathologie, Bd. 3. Witzstork, Baden-Baden 1981

Lübke, F., M. Schmidt-Gollwitzer: First experience with hysteroscopy. Fortschr. Endosc. 4 (1973) 181

Lübke, F.: Erste Erfahrungen mit der Hysteroskopie. Geburtsh. Frauenheilk. 34 (1974) 387

Lübke, F.: The diagnostic value of intrauterine causes for sterility and infertility, using hysteroscopy. Presented at the VIII World Congress on Fertility and Sterility. Buenos Aires, Nov. 3-9, 1974

Lübke, F.: Über den diagnostischen Wert der Hysteroskopie. Arch. Gynäkol. 219 (1975) 255

Lübke, F.: Kritische Bemerkungen zur Hysteroskopie. Acta Endosc. Radiocinematogr. 7 (1977) 49

Lübke, F.: Hysteroscopy as a routine clinical method. In H. Van der Pas, B. Van Herendael, D. Van Lith, C. Keith: Hysteroscopy. MTP Press, Boston (1983) (p. 95)

Lübke, F.: Importance of hysteroscopy as a clinical method for examination. In A.M. Siegler, H.J. Lindemann: Hysteroscopy: Principles and Practice. Lippincott, Philadelphia 1984 (p. 302)

Lübke, F., H.J. Hindenburg: Hysteroscopy as an examination method in sterility. In A.M. Siegler, H.J. Lindemann: Hysteroscopy: Principles and Practice. Lippincott, Philadelphia 1984, (p. 173)

Lübke, F.: Principles and practice of hysteroscopy. Acta Europ. Fertil. 17 (1986) 413

Lueken, R.P., H.J. Lindemann: Diagnosis and treatment of lost IUD's using CO₂-hysteroscopy. Endoscopy 9 (1977) 119

Lueken, R.P., H.J. Lindemann: Therapeutic possibilities with hysteroscopy. Endoscopy 10 (1978) 232

Lueken, R.P.: Position und Kinetik von Intrauterinpessaren. Keitumer Kreis 2 (1980) 4

Lueken, R.P.: Photographic documentation of hysteroscopy. In H. Van der Pas, B. Van Herendael, D.A.F. Van Lith, L. Keith: Hysteroscopy: MTP Press, Boston 1983 (p. 49)

Macdonald, R., J. Phipps, A. Singer: Endometrial ablation: a safe procedure. Gynecol. Endoscopy 1 (1992) 7

Madsen, P.O., O.E. Knuth, L.V. Wagenbrecht: Über die Spülflüssigkeiten und ihre Absorption während der transurethralen Prostataresektion. Urologe 8 (1969) 309

Madsen, P.O., R.E. Madsen: Clinical and experimental evaluation of different irrigation fluids for transurethral surgery. Investig. Urol. 3 (1965) 122

Magos, A.L., R. Baumann, A.C. Turnbull: Transcervical resection of endometrium in women with menorrhagia. Brit. ed. J. 298 (1989) 1209

Magos, A.L., R. Baumann, G.M. Lockwood, A.C. Turnbull: Experience with the first 250 endometrial resections for menorrhagia. Lancet 337 (1991) 1074

Malter, A.: Angewandte Leistungserfassung von Hysteroskopie und vaginaler Sonographie in der Praxis. Vortrag: 161 Tagung der Mittelrheinischen Gesellschaft für Gynäkologie und Geburtshilfe, Heidelberg, Juni 1989

Mangar, D., J.I. Gerson, R.M. Constantine, V. Lenzi: Pulmonary edema and coagulopathy due to Hyskon (32 % dextran-70) administration. Anesth. Analg. 68 (1989) 686

March, C.M., R. Israel: Hysteroscopic management of recurrent abortion caused by septate uterus. Am. J. Obstet. Gynecol. 156 (1987) 834

Marleschki, V.: Moderne Cervicoscopie und Hysteroscopie. Abhandlungen der Deutschen Akademie der Wissenschaften zu Berlin. Akademie-Verlag, Berlin 3 (1966) 421

Marleschki, V.: Die moderne Zervikoskopie und Hysteroskopie. Zbl. Gynäkol. 88 (1966) 637

Marleschki, V.: Ein weiterer Schritt in der Frühdiagnose des Intrazervikal- und Korpuskarzinoms. Krebsarzt 21 (1966) 159

Marleschki, V.: Hysteroskopische Feststellung der spontanen Perfusionsschwankungen am menschlichen Endometrium. Zbl. Gynäkol. 90 (1968) 1094

Marleschki, V.: Das Universal-Hysteroskop nach Marleschki. Urania 6 (1971) 34

Marleschki, V.: Contact hysteroscopy with the universal 4 mm hysteroscope. In A.M. Siegler, H.J. Lindemann: Hysteroscopy: Principles and Practice. Lippincott, Philadelphia 1984 (p. 58)

Marty, R.: Carbon dioxide hysteroscopy without anesthesia in 478 patients. In A.M. Siegler, H.J. Lindemann: Hysteroscopy: Principles and Practice. Lippincott, Philadelphia 1984

Marty, R.: Hysteroscopy necessary before IUD. Acta Europ. Fertil. 17 (1986) 449

Mazzon, I., V Scotto, M.L. Guidi, G. Vittori, G. Ricci, G. Crisci, A. Pignanelli: Outpatient hysteroscopy in the diagnosis of neoplastic and preneoplastic lesions of the endometrium. Eur. J. Gynecol. Oncol. 3 (1988) 261

Mencaglia, L., C. Tantini, M. Colafranceschi, G. Taddei, G. Scarselli: Hysteroscopic evulation of precancerous endometrial lesions. In H. Van der Pas, B. Van Herendael, D. Van Lith, C. Keith: Hysteroscopy. MTP Press, Boston 1983 (p. 129)

Mencaglia, L. F. Branconi, G. Scarselli, F. Locatelli, L. Savino, E. Chelo, M. Marchionni: Microcolposcopy in the diagnosis and management of cervical intraepithelial neoplasia. Europ. J. Gynecol. Oncol. 4 (1983) 216

Mencaglia, L.: Hysteroscopy versus curettage. Vortrag: Second World Congress on Hysteroscopy. Berlin 1985

Mencaglia, L., A. Perino: Diagnostic hysteroscopy today. Acta Europ. Fertil. 17 (1986) 431

Mencaglia, L., G. Ricci, A. Perino, E. Cittadini, E. Catinella: Hysteroscopic chorionic villi sampling: a new approach. Acta Europ. Fertil. 17 (1986) 491

Mencaglia, L., A. Perino, J.E. Hamou: Hysteroscopy in peri-menopausal and postmenopausal women with abnormal uterine bleeding. J. Reprod. Med. 32 (1987) 577

Mencaglia, L.: Endometrial cytology: six years of experience. Diagn. Cytopathol. 3 (1987) 185

Mencaglia, L., M. Colafranceschi, A.G. Gordon, H. Lindemann: Is hysteroscopy of value in the investigation of female infertility? Acta Europ. Fertil. 19 (1988) 239

Menken, F.C.: Fortschritte der gynäkologischen Endoskopie. In L. Demling, R. Allenjahn: Fortschritte der Endoskopie. Schattauer, Stuttgart 1969

Menken, F.C.: Ein neues Verfahren mit Vorrichtung zur Hysteroskopie. Endoscopy 3 (1971) 200

Menken, F.C.: Hysteroskopie: Methode praxisreif. Selecta 25 (1972) 2459

Menken, F.C.: Endoscopy procedures and their combined application in gynecology. J. Reprod. Med. 12 (1974) 250

Menken, F.C.: Microendoscopy of the uterine cervix. Geburtsh. Frauenheilk. 41 (1981) 192

Mergui, J.L., J. Salat-Baroux: Section des cloisons uterines sous hysteroscopie. Presse Med. 18 (1989) 488

Mestwerdt, W., P. Kranzfelder: Neue diagnostische Möglichkeiten beim Endometriumcarcinom und seinen Vorstufen. Gynäkologie 16 (1983) 87

Mestwerdt, W.: Moderatorenbericht: Früherkennung des Endometrium-Ca. Arch. Gynäkol. 235 (1983)

Mikulicz-Radecki, F., A. Freund: Das Tubenhysteroskop und seine diagnostische Verwendung bei Sterilität, Sterilisierung und Tubenerkrankungen. Arch. Gynäkol. 123 (1927) 68

Mikulicz-Radecki, F., A. Freund: Ein neues Hysteroskop und seine praktische Anwendung in der Gynäkologie. Geburtsh. u. Gynäkol. 92 (1928) 12

Mikulicz-Radecki, F.: Weitere Erfahrungen mit der Hysteroskopie insbesondere beim Stadium des Endometriums. Zbl. Gynäkol. 53 (1929) 258

Mohr, J., H.J. Lindemann: Hysteroscopy as a diagnostic method in female sterility. Fortschr. Androl. 3 (1974) 102

Mohr, J., H.J. Lindemann: Vergleichende Resultate zwischen CO_2-Hysteroskopie, Hysterosalpingographie und Histologie. Arch. Gynäkol. 219 (1975) 256

Mohr, J., H.J. Lindemann: CO_2-Hysteroskopie, eine Methode zur Entfernung okkulter Intrauterinpessare. Arch. Gynäkol. 224 (1977) 31

Mohr, J., H.J. Lindemann: Transuterine Tubensterilisation per Hysteroskop mit einem Gewebekleber. Acta Endosc. Radiocinematogr. 7 (1977) 47

Mohri, T.: Our 25 years' experience with endoscopes. Jinmu Shobo, Tokyo 1975

Mohri, T., C. Mohri, F. Yamadori: Tubaloscope: Flexible glassfiber endoscope for intratubal observation, Endoscopy 226 (1979)

Molnár, B.G., J.A.M. Broadbent, A.L. Magos: Fluid overload risk score for endometrial resection. Gynecol. Endoscopy 1 (1992) 133

Moulay, A., M. Zahl: La migration abdominale des dispositifs intrautdrins. A propos de quatre cas extraits par cœlioscopie. Sem. Hop. Paris 59 (1983) 2905

Naber, K., K. Möhring: Zum Problem der Spülflüssigkeitseinschwemmung bei der transurethralen Prostataresektion. Urologe 12 (1973) 206

Nagel, T.C., R.A. Kopher, G.E. Tagatz, T. Okagaki, D.C. Brooker: Tubal reflux of endometrial tissue during hysteroscopy. In A.M. Siegler, H.J. Lindemann: Hysteroscopy: Principles and Practice. Lippincott, Philadelphia 1984 (p. 145)

Neis, K.J., N.K. Schöndorf, V.J. Uhl, A. Veldung: Die Aktinomykose des weiblichen Genitaltraktes bei IUD-Trägerinnen. Geburtsh. Frauenheilk. 42 (1982) 48

Neis, K.J., A.K.J. Brachetti: Die Bedeutung der histologischen Klassifizierung bei der Prognose des Ovarialcarcinoms. Arch. Gynecol. Obstet. 232 (1982) 263

Neis, K.J., N.K. Schöndorf: Zur Problematik der präoperativen Diagnostik des Zervixbefalls beim Endometriumkarzinom. Geburtsh. Frauenheilk. 43 (1983) 589

Neis, K.J., H. Hepp: Kontaktmikrokolpohysteroskopie: kritische Bilanz erster Erfahrungen. In H.J. Lindemann: Moderatorenbericht: gynäkologische und geburtshilfliche Endoskopie. Arch. Gynäkol. 235 (1983) 11

Neis, K.J., M. Bitsch, N.K. Schöndorf: Zur Treffsicherheit der Vaginalzytologie beim Adenokarzinom des Endometriums. Geburtsh. Frauenheilk. 44 (1984) 291

Neis, K.J., M. Bitsch, H. Hepp: Ergebnisse einer kombinierten hysteroskopischen und zytologischen Diagnostik zur Erfassung pathologischer Veränderungen des Endometriums. In R. Kaiser: Klinische Forschung in der Gynäkologie und Geburtshilfe. Thieme, Stuttgart 1985 (S. 33)

Neis, K.J., M. Bitsch, N.K. Schöndorf: Möglichkeiten der differentialzytologischen Beurteilung von Endometriumsabstrichen. Arch. Gynäkol. 238 (1985) 600

Neis, K.J., M. Bitsch, H. Hepp: Die ambulante hysteroskopische und bioptische Abklärung der Postmenopausenblutung eine Alternative zur konventionellen Abrasio. In H.J. Lindemann: Moderatorenbericht: Gynäkologische und geburtshilfliche Endoskopie. Arch. Gynäkol. 238 (1985) 11

Neis, K., H. Hepp: The accuracy of combined hysteroscopy and line biopsy under ambulatory conditions. Acta Europ. Fertil. 17 (1986) 445

Nesbit, R.M., S.I. Glickmann: The use of glycine solution as an irrigating medium during transurethral resection. J. Urol. 59 (1948): 1212

Neuwirth, R.S.: A new technique for and additional experience with hysteroscopic resection of submucous fibroids. Am. J. Obstet. Gynecol. 131 (1978) 91

Neuwirth, R.S., R.V Levine: Evaluation of a method of hysteroscopy with the use of 30 % dextran. Am. J. Obstet. Gynecol. 114 (1972) 696

Neuwirth, R.S., H.K. Amin: Excision of submucos fibroids with hysteroscopic control. Am. J. Obstet. Gynecol. 126 (1976) 95

Neuwirth, R.S.: Operative hysteroscopy. In V. Albano, E. Cittadini: Endoscopia Gynecologica. Cofese, Palermo 1981

Neuwirth, R.S.: Hysteroscopic management of symptomatic submucous fibroids. Obstet. Gynecol. 62 (1983) 509

Neuwirth, R.S.: Hysteroscopic resection of submucous fibroids. In A.M. Siegler, H.J. Lindemann: Hysteroscopy: Principles and Practice. Lippincott, Philadelphia 1984

Ng, A.B.P., J.W. Reagan, R. Cechner: The precursors of endometrial cancer: a study of their cellular manifestations. Acta cytol. 17 (1973) 439

Ng, A.B.P.: The cellular detection of endometrial cancer and its precursors. Gynecol. Oncol. 2 (1974) 162

Ng, A.B.P., R. Richart: Vorstufen des Corpuscarcinoms. Klin. J. 9 (1983) 48

Nitze, M.: Eine neue Betrachtungs- und Untersuchungsmethode für Harnröhre, Harnblase und Rectum. Wien. med. Wschr. 29 (1879) 650

Norlén, H.: Isotonic solutions of mannitol, sorbitol and glycine and distilled water as irrigating fluids during transurethral resection of the prostate and calculation of irrigating fluid influx. Scand. J. Urol. Nephrol. (1985) Suppl. No. 96

Noss, U., K.J. Neis, M. Bitsch, H. Hepp: Die Bedeutung des Gestagentests zur Verlaufskontrolle nach glandulär-zystischer Hyperplasie. Arch. Gynäkol. 238 (1985) 757

Ohkawa, K., R. Ohkawa: Hysteromicroscopy. In A.M. Siegler, H.J. Lindemann: Hysteroscopy: Principles and Practice. Lippincott, Philadelphia 1984 (p. 84)

Ortner, A., J. Klammern A. Bichler, G. Weiser, W. Kalkschmid, W. Geier: Prüfung von zwei Methoden (Pistolet und Jet-washing) zur Gewebegewinnung aus dem Cavum uteri. Geburtsh. Frauenheilk. 38 (1978) 88

Otte, C.: Experimentelle Untersuchungen zur potentiellen Einsatzmöglichkeit des Nd:YAG-Lasers zur hysteroskopischen Tubensterilisation. Dissertation Homburg/Saar 1992

Ovassapian, A., C.W. Joshi, E.A. Brunner: Visual disturbances: An unusual symptom of transurethral prostatic resection reaction. Anaesthesiology 57 (1982) 332

Pace, S., P. Franceschini, M. Figliolini: Miomectomia per via isteroscopia. Minerva Ginecol. 44 (1992) 623

Palmer, R., R. Michon: L'hystéroscopie cervicale. Gynécol. et Obstét. 42 (1942) 134

Palmer, R.: Un nouvel hystéroscope. Bull. Féd. Soc. Gynécol. Obstét. franç. 9 (1957) 300

Pantaleoni, D.: An endoscopic examination of the cavity of the womb. Med. Press 8 (1869) 26

Parent, B., C. Toubas: Une nouvelle technique d'exploration de la cavité utérine: 14 hystérocopies de contact. Concours méd. 95 (1973) 1635

Parent, B.: Hysteroscopie de contact. D.E.P., Paris 1976

Parent, B., J. Barbot, B. Doerler: Hystéroscopie de contact. Nouv. Presse méd. 6 (1977) 113

Parent, B., H. Guedj, J. Barbot, P. Nodarian: Hystéroscopie Panoramique. Maloine, Paris 1985

Pellicer, A.: Hysteroscopy in the infertile woman. Obstet. Gynecol. Clin. N. Amer. 15 (1988) 99

Perino, A., E. Catinella, G. Comparetto, R. Venezia, P. Candela, C. Cimino, C. Zangara, L. Mencaglia: Hysteroscopic metroplasty: the role of ultrasound in the diagnosis and monitoring of patients with uterine septa. Acta Europ. Fertil. 18 (1987) 349

Peterson, H.B., J.F. Hulka, J.M. Phillips: American Association of Gynecologic Laparoscopists 1988 membership survey on operative hysteroscopy. J. Reprod. Med. 35 (1990) 590

Petrucco, O.M., A. Gillespie: The neodymium:YAG laser and the resectoscope for the treatment of menorrhagia. Med. J. Aust. 154 (1991) 518

Phipps, J.H., B.V. Lewis, M.V. Prior, T. Roberts: Experimental and clinical studies with radiofrequency-induced thermal ablation for functional menorrhagia. Obstet. Gynecol. 76 (1990) 876

Popp, L.W., R.P. Lueken, W. Mueller-Holve, H.J. Lindemann: Gynecologic endosonography: initial experiences. Ultraschall medicus 4 (1983) 92

Popp, L.W., R.P. Lueken: Hysterosonography: a new approach for extending endoscopic observation. In A.M. Siegler, H.J. Lindemann: Hysteroscopy: Principles and Practice. Lippincott, Philadelphia 1984

Popp, L.W.: Endosonographische Methoden in Geburtshilfe und Gynäkologie. In L.W. Popp: Gynäkologische Endosonographie. Klemke, Quickborn 1986

Pyper, R.J.D., A.D. Haeri: A review of 80 endometrial resections for menorrhagia. Br. J. Obstet. Gynaecol. 98 (1991) 1049

Rancke, F., N. Schmeller, M. Albrecht: Zusatz von Äthylalkohol zur Spülflüssigkeit – Überwachung der Einschwemmung bei transurethralen Prostataresektionen. Anaesthesist 41 (1992) 324

Rath, W: Intracervical prostaglandin-gel application to facilitate cervical dilatation prior to hysteroscopy. Vortrag: Second World Congress on Hysteroscopy, Berlin 1985

Reagan, J.W., A.B.P. Ng: The cells of uterine adenocarinoma, Monographs in clinical cytology, Vol. 1. Karger, Basel 1973

Reagan, J.W.: Can screening for endometrial cancer be justified. Acta cytol. 24 (1980) 87

Reed, T.P., R. Erb: Hysteroscopic tubal occlusion with silicone rubber. Obstet. Gynecol. 61 (1983) 388

Reich, H., T. Vancaillie, R.M. Soederstrom: Electrical techniques. In: Martin, D.C., G.L. Holtz, C.J. Levinson, R.M. Soederstrom (eds) Manual of endoscopy. Port City Press (1990) 105

Renaer, M., L. Vandervoort, P. Ide, F. De Wolf: Investigation of patients with postmenopausal bleeding. In H. Van der Pas, B. Ide, P. Van Herendael, D. Van Lith, C. Keith: Hysteroscopy. MTP Press, Boston 1983 (p. 121)

Riedel, H.J., K. Semm: Das postpelviskopische (laparoskopische) subphrenische Schmerzsyndrom. Arch. Gynäkol. 20 (1979) 228

Riehm, S., U. Haselbach, K.J. Neis, G. Basten: Immunhistochemische Darstellung des Östrogen- und Progesteronrezeptors am Endometrium postmenopausaler Frauen. Ber. Gynäkol. Geburtsh. 7 (1986) 500

Rimkus, V., K. Semm: Sterilization by carbon dioxide hysteroscopy. In J.J. Sciarra, J.C. Butler, J.J. (eds) Spiedel: Hysteroscopy Sterilization. Intercontinental Medical Book Corporation, New York (1974) (p. 75)

Rimkus, V., K. Semm: Die Schwachstromkoagulation als Methode der Sterilisation unter hysteroskopischer Kontrolle. Arch. Gynäkol. 219 (1975) 49

Roesch, R.P., R.K. Stoelting, K.E. Lingemann, R.J. Kahnoski, D.J. Backes, S.A. Gephardt: Ammonia toxicity resulting from glycine absorption during a transurethral resection of the prostate. Anaesthesiology 58 (1983) 577

Rohde, D.: Zytologische Diagnostik des Endometriumkarzinoms durch vaginale und intrauterine Materialentnahme. MD-GBK 45 (1985) 19

Rubin, I.C.: Uterine endoscopy, endometroscopy with the aid of uterine insufflation. Am. J. Obstet. Gynecol. 10 (1925) 313

Ryder, K.W., J.F. Olsen, R.J. Kahnoski, R.C. Karn, T.O. Oei: Hyperammonemia after transurethral resection of the prostate: A report of 2 cases. Journal of Urology 132 (1984) 995

Salat-Baroux, J., J. Hamou: La microcolposcopie, une nouvelle méthode, son application en gynécologie. Méd. Hyg. 38 (1980) 1696

Salat-Baroux, J., J.E. Hamou, G. Maillard, A. Chouraqui, P. Verges: Complications from microhysteroscopy. In A.M. Siegler, H.J. Lindemann: Hysteroscopy: Principles and Practice. Lippincott, Philadelphia 1984 (p. 112)

Sauter, Th.: Aktueller Stand der Transvaginalsonographie, TW Gynäkologie 2 (1989) 21-29

Scarselli, G., C. Tantini, L. Mencaglia, E. Chelo, A. Gargiulo: Microhysteroscopy and infertility. In H. Van der Pas, B. Van Herendael, D.A.F. van Lith, L. Keith: Hysteroscopy. MTP Press, Boston 1983 (p. 151)

Scarselli, G., L. Mencaglia, M. Colafranceschi, G. Taddei, F. Branconi, C. Tartini: The standardization of morphologic precursors of endometrial adenocarcinoma by microhysteroscopy. In A.M. Siegler, H.J. Lindemann: Hysteroscopy: Principles and Practice. Lippincott, Philadelphia 1984 (p. 151)

Schachter A., A. Beckerman, C. Bahary, S.J. Joel-Cohen: The value of cytology in the diagnosis of endometrial pathology. Acta cytol. 24 (1980) 149

Schack, L.: Unsere Erfahrungen mit der Hysteroskopie. Zbl. Gynäkol. 60 (1936) 1810

Schmidt-Matthiesen, H.: Die Hysteroskopie als klinische Routinemethode. Geburtsh. Frauenheilk. 26 (1966) 1498

Schneider, M.L.: Möglichkeiten und Grenzen eines zytologischen Früherkennungsprogramms beim Endometriumkarzinom. Geburtsh. Frauenheilk. 45 (1985) 831

Schöndorf, N.K.: Grundlagen, Ergebnisse und klinischer Stellenwert der differentialzytologischen Diagnostik bei Mammaerkrankungen. Habil. Saarland 1982

Schroeder, T.M., P.A. Poulakkainen, J. Hahl, J. Ramo: Fatal air embolism as a complication of laser induced hyperthermia. Lasers Surg. Med. 9 (1989) 183

Schulz, K.D.: New concepts of adjuvant drug treatment in endometrial cancer. Vortrag: 3rd International Symposium on Endometrial Cancer. Marburg 1986

Schweppe, K.W., H. Wagner, F.K. Beller: Zur Diagnostik und Therapie okkulter Intrauterinpessare bei eingetretener Schwangerschaft. Geburtsh. Frauenheilk. 42 (1982) 829

Seinera, P., S. Maccario, L. Visentin, A. Di Gregorio: Hysteroscopy in an IVF-ER program. Clinical experience with 360 infertile patients. Acta Obstet. Gynecol. Scand. 67, 2 (1988) 135

Seki, M., L. Mettler, K. Semm: Comparison of fluid hysteroscopy and CO_2-hysteroscopy. Endoscopy 14 (1982) 141

Semm, K.: Transabdominale oder transvaginale Eileitersterilisation mit einer neuen Koagulationszange. Endoscopy 6 (1970) 40

Semm, K., V. Rimkus: Technische Bemerkungen zur CO_2-Hysteroskopie. Geburtsh. Frauenheilk. 34 (1974) 329

Semm, K.: Pelviskopie und Hysteroskopie. Farbatlas und Lehrbuch. Schattauer, Stuttgart 1976

Semm, K.: Kontakt-hysteroskopische Fetoskopie. Gynäkol. Prax. 2 (1978) 369

Semm, K., H.H. Riedel: The clinical value of hysteroscopy. In A.M. Siegler, H.J. Lindemann: Hysteroscopy: Principles and Practice. Lippincott, Philadelphia 1984 (p. 310)

Serden, S.P., P.G. Brooks: Treatment of abnormal uterine bleeding with the gynecologic resectoscope. J. Reprod. Med. 36 (1991): 697

Siegler, A.M.: A comparison of gas and liquid for hysteroscopy. J. reprod. Med. 15 (1975) 73

Siegler, A.M.: Hysterography and hysteroscopy in the infertile patient. Obstet. Gynecol. 18 (1977) 143

Siegler, A.M.: Risks and complications of hysteroscopy. In H. Van der Pas, B. Van Lith, C. Keith: Hysteroscopy. MTP Press, Boston 1983 (p. 75)

Siegler, A.M.: Panoramic CO_2-hysteroscopy. Clin. Obstet. Gynecol. 26 (1983) 242

Siegler, A.M.: The quest for a hysteroscopic method of sterilization. In A.M. Siegler, H.J. Lindemann: Hysteroscopy: Principles and Practice. Lippincott, Philadelphia 1984 (p. 239)

Siegler, A.M.: Adverse effects. In A.M. Siegler, H.J. Lindemann: Hysteroscopy: Principles and Practice. Lippincott, Philadelphia 1984

Siegler, A.: Therapeutic hysteroscopy. Acta Europ. Fertil. 17 (1986) 467

Siegler, A.M., R.F. Valle: Therapeutic hysteroscopic procedures. Fertil. Steril. 50 (1988) 685

Silander, T.: Hysteroscopy through a transparent rubber ballon. Surg. Gynecol. Obstet. 114 (1962) 125

Snowden, E.U., J.C. Jarrett, M.Y. Dawood: Comparison of diagnostic accuracy of laparoscopy, hysteroscopy and hysterosalpingography in evaluation of female infertility. Fertil. Steril. 41 (1984) 709

Soost, H.J., S. Bauer: Gynäkologische Zytodiagnostik. Lehrbuch und Atlas. Thieme, Stuttgart 1980

Soost, H.J.: Möglichkeiten der Früherkennung des Endometriumcarcinoms. Geburtsh. Frauenheilk. 42 (1982) 899

Sorensen, S.S.: Hysteroscopic evaluation and endocrinological aspects of women with mullerian anomalies and oligomenorrhea. Int. J. Fertil. 32 (1987) 445

Stelmachow, J.: The role of hysteroscopy in gynecologic oncology. Gynecol. Oncol. 14 (1982) 392

Stock, R.J., A. Kanbour: Prehysterectomy curettage. Obstet. Gynecol. 45 (1975) 537

Stoeckel, W: Lehrbuch der Gynäkologie, 4. Aufl. Hirzel, Leipzig 1933 (S. 103)

Sugimoto, O.: Hysteroscopic diagnosis of endometrial carcinoma. A report of fifty-three cases examined at the Woman's Clinic of Kyoto University Hospital. Am. J. Obstet. Gynecol. 121 (1975) 105

Sugimoto, O., T. Ushiroyama, Y. Fukuda: Diagnostic and therapeutic hysteroscopy for traumatic intrauterine adhesions. In A.M. Siegler, H.J. Lindemann: Hysteroscopy: Principles and Practice. Lippincott, Philadelphia 1984

Sugimoto, O., T. Ushiroyama, Y. Fukuda: Diagnostic hysteroscopy for endometrial carcinoma. In A.M. Siegler, H.J. Lindemann: Hysteroscopy: Principles and Practice. Lippincott, Philadelphia 1984 (p. 157)

Suzuki, A., H. Tahara, H. Okamura: Hysteroscopic diagnosis of malignant mixed müllerian tumor of the corpus uteri. Gynecol. Oncol. 15 (1983) 350

Surrey, M.W., S. Aronberg: Hysteroscopic diagnosis of abnormal uterine bleeding: a clinical study. In A.M. Siegler, H.J. Lindemann: Hysteroscopy: Principles and Practice. Lippincott, Philadelphia 1984

Sweeney, W.J.: Hysterosalpingography. Obstet. Gynecol. 11 (1958) 640

Swolin, K., M. Rosencrantz: Laparoscopy vs. hysterosalpingography in sterility investigation. A comparative study. Fertil. Steril. 23 (1972) 270

Tadese, A., K. Wamsteker: Evaluation of 24 patients with IUD-related problems: hysteroscopic findings. Europ. J. Obstet. Gynecol. 19 (1985) 37

Takashima, E.: Usefulness of hysteroscopy for detection of cancer in the endocervical canal. Nippon Sanka Fujinka Gakkai Zasshi 37 (1985) 2401

Taylor, P.J.: Correlations in infertility: symptomatology, hysterosalpingography, laparoscopy and hysteroscopy. J. Reprod. Med. 18 (1977) 339

Taylor, P.J., D.C. Cumming: Hysteroscopy in 100 patients. Fertil. Steril. 31 (1979) 301

Taylor, P.J., D.C. Cumming, P.J. Hill: Significance of intrauterine adhesions detected hysteroscopically in eumenorrheic infertile women and role of antecedent curettage in their formation. Am. J. Obstet. Gynecol. 139 (1981) 239

Taylor, P.J., G. Graham: Is diagnostic curettage harmful to women with unexplained infertility? Brit. J. Obstet. Gynaecol. 89 (1982) 296

Taylor, P.J., A. Leader, R.E. Georg: Combined laparoscopy and hysteroscopy in the investigation of infertility. In A.M. Siegler, H.J. Lindemann: Hysteroscopy: Principles and Practice. Lippincott, Philadelphia 1984 (p. 207)

Taylor, P.J., D. Lewinthal, A. Leader, H.A. Pattinson: A comparison of Dextran 70 with carbon dioxide as the distention medium for hysteroscopy in patients with infatility or requesting reversal of a prior tubal sterilization. Fertil. Steril. 47 (1987) 861

Thom, M.H., P.J. White, R.M. Williams et al.: Prevention and treatment of endometrial disease in climateric women receiving estrogen therapy. Lancet (1979), 455

Toro-Calzada, R.J., A.M. Garcia-Luna, A.D. Manterola: Histeroscopia en infertilidad. Ginecol. Obstet. Mex. 60 (1992) 267

Townsend, D.E., D.R. Ostergard, D.Jr. Mischell et al.: Abnormal Papanicolaou smears. Am. J. Obstet. Gynecol. 108 (1970) 429

Trimbos-Kemper, T.C., B.T. Veering: Anaphylactic shock from intracavitary 32 % dextran 70 during hysteroscopy. Fertil. Steril. 51 (1989) 1053

Trunninger, B.: Elektrolytprobleme des urologischen Patienten. Aktuelle Urologie 7 (1976) 1

Tulandi, T., J. Hilton: Effects of intraperitoneal 32% dextran-70 on blood coagulation and serum electrolytes. J. Reprod. Med. 30 (1985) 431

Valle, J.A., A.S. Lifchez, J. Moise: A simpler technique for reduction of uterine septum. Fertil. Steril. 56 (1991) 1001

Valle, R.F., D.W. Freeman: Hysteroscopy in the management of the lost intrauterine device. Adv. Plan. Parent. 10 (1975) 164

Valle, R.F., J.J. Sciarra, D.W. Freeman: Hysteroscopic removal of intrauterine devices with missing filaments. Obstet. Gynecol. 49 (1977) 55

Valle, R.F., J.J. Sciarra: Hysteroscopy for gynecologic diagnosis. Clin. Obstet. Gynecol. 26 (1983) 253

Valle, R.F.: Hysteroscopy in the evaluation of female infertility. Am. J. Obstet. Gynecol. 137 (1980) 425

Valle, R.F.: Hysteroscopic evaluation of patients with abnormal uterine bleeding. Surg. Gynecol. Obstet. 153 (1981) 521

Valle, R.F., J.J. Sciarra: Hysteroscopic treatment of intrauterine adhesions. In A.M. Siegler, H.J. Lindemann: Hysteroscopy: Principles and Practice. Lippincott, Philadelphia 1984 (p. 193)

Valle, R.F: Therapeutic hysteroscopy in infertility. Int. J. Fertil. 29 (1984) 143

Valle, R.F.: Indications. In A.M. Siegler, H.J. Lindemann: Hysteroscopy: Principles and Practice. Lippincott, Philadelphia 1984 (p. 21)

Valle, R.F.: Future growth and development of hysteroscopy. Obstet. Gynecol. Clin. N. Amer. 15, 1 (1988) 111-126

Valle, R.F., J.J. Sciarra: Intrauterine adhesions: hysteroscopic diagnosis, classification, treatment and reproductive outcome. Am. J. Obstet. Gynecol. 158 (1988) 1459

Vancaillie, T.G., E. De Muylder: Hysteroscopic evalution of hormonal influence on the endometrium. In H. Van der Pas, B. Van Herendael, D. Van Lith, C. Keith: Hysteroscopy. MTP Press, Boston 1983 (p. 101)

Vancaillie, T.G., C.A. Eddy, L. Laufe: A new method of transcervical female sterilization: preliminary results in rabbits. Fertil. Steril. 51 (1989) 335

Vancaillie, T.G.: Electrocoagulation of the endometrium with the ball-end resectoscope. Obstet. Gynecol. 74 (1989) 425

Van Herendael, B.J.: Hysteroscopy in subfertility. In H. Van der Pas, B. Van Herendael, D.A.F. Van Lith, L. Keith: Hysteroscopy. MTP Press, Boston 1985 (p. 193)

Van Herendael, B.J., M.J. Stevens, A. Flakiewicz-Kula, C. Hansch: Dating of the endometrium by microhysteroscopy. Gynecol. Obstet. Invest. 24, 2 (1987) 114-118

Van der Pas, H.: Outpatient hysteroscopy: an acquisition for the gynecologist? T. soc. Geneesk. 13 (1979) 867

Van der Pas, H.: Die ambulante Hysteroskopie als Untersuchungsmethode in der Gynäkologie. Keitumer Kreis 1980

Van der Pas, H., B.J. Van Herendael: Hysteroscopy Slide Atlas. Palfijin Foundation, Antwerpen 1982

Van der Pas, H.: Hysteroscopy as an out-patient procedure. In A.M. Siegler, H.J. Lindemann: Hysteroscopy: Principles and Practice. Lippincott, Philadelphia 1984 (p. 104)

Van der Pas, H.: Hysteroscopic retrieval of IUD in first trimester of pregnancy. Acta Obstet. Gynecol. Scand 64 (1985)

Van der Pas, H.: Hysteroscopic treatment of early pregnancy conceived despite intrauterine contraception. Acta Europ. Fertil. 17 (1986) 481

Van der Spruy, Z.M., A.G. Fieggan, M.A. Wood, C.A. Piennaar: The short term use of luteinizing hormone releasing analogues in uteri e fibroids. Hormon Res. 32 (1989) 137

Van Deyk, K., R. Harzmann, R. Schorer, K.-H. Bichler: Einschwemmung von Spülflüssigkeit bei transurethraler Prostataresektion – Impedanzcardiographische Untersuchungen. Anaesthesist 30 (1981) 549

Van Roessel, J., K. Wamsteker, N. Exalto: Sonographic investigation of the uterus artificial uterine cavity distention. ICU (1987) 439-450

Vercellini, R, L. Fedele, L. Arcaini, M.T. Rognoni, G.B. Candiani: Value of intrauterine device insertion and estrogen administration after hysteroscopic metroplasty. J. Reprod. Med. 34, 7 (1989) 447

Wagner, H., K.W Schweppe, H.L. Kronholz, et al.: Möglichkeiten der Extraktion von Intrauterinpessaren bei eingetretener Schwangerschaft. Med. Welt 31 (1980) 1317

Wagner, H.: Lost IUD. Keitumer Kreis 1980

Wagner, H., K.W. Schweppe, F.K. Beller: Fragmentation von Intrauterinpessaren als Komplikation bei der Extraktion. Geburtsh. Frauenheilk. 43 (1983) 123

Wagner, H.: Diagnosis and treatment of complications of intrauterine contraceptive devices. In H. Van der Pas, B. Van Herendael, D. Van Lith, C. Keith: Hysteroscopy. MTP Press, Boston 1983 (p. 185)

Wagner, H., K.W. Schweppe: The influence of intrauterine device displacement on the pregnancy date. In A.M. Siegler, H.J. Lindemann: Hysteroscopy: Principles and Practice. Lippincott, Philadelphia 1984

Wallwiener, D., D. Pollmann, S. Rimbach, W. Stolz, C. Sohn, G. Bastert: Operative Hysteroskopie in der Fertilitätschirurgie. Gynäkol. Prax. 17 (1993) 109

Wallwiener, D., S. Rimbach, D. Pollmann, G. Bastert: Endoskopische Präparationstechniken. In: Endoscopic surgery in gynecology, Lueken, R.P., A. Gallinat (Hrsg.), Demeter Verlag Gräfelfing (1992) 9

Wamsteker, K.: Hysteroscopic surgery. In H. Van der Pas, B. Van Herendael, D.A.F. Van Lith, L. Keith: Hysteroscopy. MTP Press, Boston 1983 (p. 165)

Wamsteker, K.: Hysteroscopic tubal sterilization with electrocoagulation and thermocoagulation. In A.M. Siegler, H.J. Lindemann: Hysteroscopy: Principles and Practice. Lippincott, Philadelphia 1984

Wamsteker, K., R.P. Lueken: Hysteroscopy in the management of abnormal uterine bleeding in 199 patients. In A.M. Siegler, H.J. Lindemann: Hysteroscopy: Principles and Practice. Lippincott, Philadelphia 1984 (p. 128)

Wamsteker, K.: Endoscopic classification of Asherman's syndrom. The Hysteroscope, Newsletter of the European Society of Hysteroscopy 4 (1989) 3

Wamsteker, K., M.H. Emanuel, J.H., de Kruif: Transcervical hysteroscopic resection of submucous fibroids for abnormal uterine bleeding: Results regarding the degree of intramural extension. Obstet. Gynecol. 82 (1993) 736

Weiss, N.S., D.R. Szekely, D.E Austin: Increasing incidence of endometrial cancer in the United States. New Engl. J. Med. 294 (1976) 1259

Wheeler, J.M., A.H. DeCherney: Office hysteroscopy. Obstet. Gynecol. Clin. N. Amer. 15, 1 (1988) 29-39

Wiedemann, R., H. Hepp: Zur differenzierten Indikationsstellung der operativen Techniken in der Reproduktionsmedizin. Mikrochirurgie, IVF und ET, GIFT und TET. Geburts. Frauenheilk. 49 (1989) 416

Wingo, P., P. Huezo, G. Rubin, H. Ory, H. Peterson: The mortality risk associated with hysterectomy. Am. J. Obstet Gynecol. 152 (1983) 803

Wiswedel, K.: Routine hysteroscopy in infertility? S. Afr. Med. J. 72, 4 (1987) 257-258

Witz, C.A., K.M. Silverburg, W.N. Burns, R.S. Schenken, D.L. Olive: Complications associated with the absorption of hysteroscopic fluid media. Fertil. Steril. 60 (1993) 745

Word, B., L.C. Gravlee, G.L. Wideman: The fallacy of simple uterine curettage. Obstet. Gynecol. 12 (1958) 642

Würfel, W., G. Krusmann, M. Rothenaicher, P. Hirsch, W. Krusmann: Pregnancy following intratubal gamete transfer by hysteroscopy. Geburtsh. Frauenheilk. 48 (1988) 401

Zbella, E.A., J. Moise, S.A. Carson: Noncardiogenic pulmonary edema secondary to intrauterine instillation of 32% dextran 70. Fertil. Steril. 43 (1985) 479

Zerwas, A., K.J. Neis: Prognostische Merkmale beim Endometriumkarzinom: histologische Neuklassifizierung und klinische Verlaufskontrolle bei 246 Patientinnen. Diss., Hamburg (1990)

Ziel, H.K.,WD. Finkle: Increased risk of endometrial carcinoma among users of conjugated estrogens. New Engl. J. Med. 293 (1975) 1167

Zipkin, B., D.L. Rosenfeld: Hysteroscopic removal of a heyman radium capsule. J. Reprod. Med. 22 (1979) 133

Zwergel, T.: Transurethrale Prostataresektion und Flüssigkeitshaushalt. Thieme Verlag, Stuttgart (1987)

Index

page numbers in *italics* refer to figures and tables

Index   119

Graafian follicle, *38, 39*
granulosa cells, 39
granulosa lutein cells, 39
grasping forceps, 4, 6, 91
gynecologic examination, bimanual, 26

H

hematometra, 100, *105*
hemolysis,, 1
histologic results, 28
hormone replacement therapy, 59
hormone treatment, 38
  adhesiolysis, 96
hydrosalpinx, rupture, 22
hyperhydration, hypotonic, 22
hypermenorrhea, 19
hyperplasia of endometrium, 61, *62-3*
hypomenorrhea, 100
hyponatremia, 22
Hyskon, 11
hysterectomy
  hysteroscopy before, 30
  laparoscopically assisted vaginal, 101
  risks, 22
  vaginal, 101
hysteroflator, 14, 15
  pneumometra maintenance, 27-8
hysterosalpingography, 88
  sterility investigation, 89
  tubal occlusion, 96
hysterosalpingram, preoperative, 97
hysteroscope, 2-3, 4-17
  3.7 x 5 mm, 33
  4-mm diameter, 33
  5-mm diameter, 32
  cervical adapter, 4, 5
  diagnostic, 4, 6
  flexible, 10
  gas inlet, 8, *9*
  introduction into cervical canal, 26
  irrigation system, 6
  laser, 6
  light cable, 4
  light source, 8, 9
  objective diameter, 4, 5, 6
  operating channel, 6
  operative, 6-8, 9, 10
  optical angle, 7
  optical plane, 4, 6
  optical system, 4
  sealing balloons, 4, *6*
  semi-flexible instruments, *7*
  shaft diameter, 6, 31
  working shaft, 5, 6
hysteroscopy
  continuous-flow, 11-13
  diagnostic, 10, *21*
  difficulties, 35
  directed biopsy combination, 79
  indications for, 18-19
  intrauterine staging of endometrial carcinoma, 81, *82*
  learning, 35-6
  morphologic verification, 65-6
  outpatient, 4
  postmenopausal, 56-7, *58,* 59, *60,* 61, *62,* 63, *64*

hysteroscopy
  premenopausal, 53, *54-5*
  side effects, 25
  streak curettage combination, 77-8, 79
  surgery, 3
  uterine bleeding, 79, 80
  uterine malformations, 87-8
  validity, 76

I

Iglesias grip, 7
impedance cardiography, 13
implantation, 20, 87
  endometrial polyps, 88
  lesions hindering, 95
  submucosal myoma, 88
infertility
  acquired uterine conditions, 88-90
  invasive therapy, 90
  investigation, 18, 86-90
  myoma, 95
  operative hysteroscopy, 95, 104
  uterine malformations, 87-8, 90
insufflators, 13
internal os, 31, 32, 33
  hysteroscopic passage, 32, *33,* 35
intracavitary pressure, 22, 28
  endometrial bleeding, 35
intrauterine adhesions, 18, 19, 88, *89,* 90, 95-7
  resection, 3
intrauterine cell collection, 67
intrauterine device (IUD)
  complications, 84
  extraction, 83
  forceps, 91
  giant cells, *71*
  infection, 71
  instruments for retrieval, 92
  lost, 18, 20, 83-4, *85*
  post-adhesiolysis, 96
  threadless, 84
intrauterine pressure
  flow rate of pumps, 12
  hydrostatic, 11
  preselection of flow, 15
  regulation, 14, 15
irrigation pumps, 12

L

labor, premature, 87, 88
lactic acidosis, 22
laparoscopy
  gamete intrafallopian transfer (GIFT), 102
  lysis of intrauterine adhesions, 96
  tubal sterilization, 101, 102
  uterine malformations, 88
  uterine septa resection, 97
laser-endoscopic technology, 3
lasers
  bare quartz glass fibers, 6
  fibers, 92-3
  sapphire tips, 92, 93
  smoke production, 6, 92

lasers
  see also argon laser; carbon dioxide, laser; Nd:YAG laser
learning hysteroscopy, 35-6
leiomyoma, 86
  enucleation, 89
  infertility assessment, 90
  miscarriage, 88-9
  submucosal, 27, 61, 80
  uterine, 21, 30
leukocyte count, 20
leuprolide acetate, 94
light
  ladder, 1
  source, 1
  see also cold-light sources
local anesthesia, 22, 23
lynestrenol, 94

M

mannitol, 11
  semi-iso-osmolar solutions, 22
menometrorrhagia, 30, 86, 98
menopausal status, 32
menopause
  endometrium, 38
  ovarian function cessation, 39
menstrual cycle, 32-3
  cervical canal patency, 32
  phase for operative hysteroscopy, 94
  stage, 34
  timing of hysteroscopy, 20
menstruation, endometrium, 44
metastases, 86
methemoglobin formation, 22
metroplasty, 97
minimally invasive surgery, 3
miscarriage
  history, 87
  leiomyoma, 88-9
mucometra, 100
müllerian duct
  misdevelopment, 97
  organ malformations, 87
müllerian tumor, mixed, 52
myoma
  infertility, 18, 95
  resection, 3, 19, 94-5, 98-9
  submucosal, 18, 19, 88, *89*
myomyectomy, hysteroscopic, 22

N

Nd:YAG laser, 3, 6, 92
  distension medium, 92, 93
  endometrial photocoagulation, 99, 100
  myoma resection, 98-9
  smoke, 6
  transuterine sterilization, 101
needle electrode, 7, 97-8
neodymium:yttrium-aluminium-garnet laser *see* Nd:YAG laser
nitrous oxide, 21
  gas embol, 22